Feminist and Anti-Psychiatry Perspectives on 'Social Anxiety Disorder'

Katie Masters

Feminist and Anti-Psychiatry Perspectives on 'Social Anxiety Disorder'

The Socially Anxious Woman

palgrave
macmillan

Katie Masters
Northampton, UK

ISBN 978-3-031-48706-4 ISBN 978-3-031-48707-1 (eBook)
https://doi.org/10.1007/978-3-031-48707-1

This Palgrave Macmillan imprint is published by the registered company Springer Nature Switzerland AG.
The registered company address is: Gewerbestrasse 11, 6330 Cham, Switzerland

Paper in this product is recyclable.

Acknowledgements

I am indebted to the seven fellow socially anxious women who all candidly shared their experiences with me: without you, this book would not have been possible. I hope I have done your stories justice.

I extend my thanks to my husband, Richard, for his enduring and unrelenting support in everything I do, and I wish to thank my brother, Oliver, for his continued reassurance and encouragement (as well as tech support!).

I am immensely grateful to Dr Nicola Smith and Professor Rosalind Gill: for their invaluable guidance, advice, and for sharing my vision of turning my doctoral thesis into a monograph.

Last, but by no means least, I wish to thank my doctoral supervisors, without whose guidance and brilliant expertise this book would not exist. Firstly, I thank Dr Emma Foster, for her unwavering kindness, support, and ability to allay my anxieties. And finally, I thank Professor Lisa Downing, for always believing in me—even, and especially, when I didn't believe in myself.

Contents

Abbreviations

APA	American Psychiatric Association
APD	Avoidant Personality Disorder
ASD	Autism Spectrum Disorder
BDD	Body Dysmorphic Disorder
CBS	Culture-Bound Syndrome
CBT	Cognitive Behavioural Therapy
CMD	Common Mental Disorder
DID	Dissociative Identity Disorder
DSM	Diagnostic and Statistical Manual of Mental Disorders
FDA	Food and Drug Administration
FSD	Female Sexual Dysfunction
GAD	Generalised Anxiety Disorder
IAPT	Improving Access to Psychological Therapies
ICD	International Classification of Diseases
MHRA	Medicines and Healthcare Products Regulatory Agency
NHS	National Health Service
NICE	National Institute for Health and Care Excellence
PMDD	Pre-menstrual Dysphoric Disorder
PMS	Pre-menstrual Syndrome
PPD	Postpartum Depression
PTSD	Post-traumatic Stress Disorder
SAD	Social Anxiety Disorder
SM	Selective Mutism
SPD	Schizoid Personality Disorder
SSRI	Selective Serotonin Reuptake Inhibitor
WHO	World Health Organization

CHAPTER 1

Introduction

'But to be happy it is essential not to be too concerned with others'.[1]

Recognising the profound and multiple ways gender socialisation has shaped my life, I found myself asking: 'Why would my experience with Social Anxiety Disorder be any different?' In a bid to find answers, I delved into modern discourses on psychiatric diagnoses, which invariably led me to popularised notions of 'chemical imbalances', 'illnesses like any other', and 'brain diseases': terms which, it seemed, had mostly been deployed by the well-meaning with the purpose of de-stigmatisation. Perhaps my being unwittingly immersed in these discourses, which pervade both popular thought and medicine, is why I bristled when reading the more absolutist claims of the 1960s anti-psychiatrists, such as Thomas S. Szasz's tenet that there is 'no such thing as mental illness'.[2] Although I found merit in the view that many 'mental illnesses' are actually 'problems in living',[3] I did not feel as though this was something I could share with people who identified with 'mental illness' labels without upsetting them: not wanting to upset people is a hallmark of my own social anxiety, to be sure.

In spite of my unease, I kept reading and slowly came to see that it is possible to critique the framework for diagnosing and treating what have been termed 'mental illnesses' without dismissing mental distress. I

K. Masters, *Feminist and Anti-Psychiatry Perspectives on 'Social Anxiety Disorder'*,
https://doi.org/10.1007/978-3-031-48707-1_1

discovered a body of work, a feminist legacy of anti-psychiatry, which theorises women's anguish without resorting to biologically reductive, 'low serotonin' explanations. This body of work privileges the importance of structural inequalities and considers the material realities of the body without recourse to arguments based on hormones or reproductive processes. Reading analyses of other gendered psychiatric diagnoses which take this approach, such as on Eating Disorders[4] and Depression,[5] I asked myself: 'Why had nobody yet applied this to women's social anxiety (disorder)?'

Overview of the Book

My mission in writing this book is to expose the degree to which cultural values, namely norms of femininity, are implicit in the psychiatric diagnosis 'Social Anxiety Disorder' (SAD)[6] in women. In so doing, the status of the socially anxious woman's experience as 'disordered' is called into question. The research on which this book is premised finds a place within a broad field of critical work, informed by Michel Foucault and others, which shows how medicine broadly, and psychiatry in particular, have become authority discourses in modernity. The rise of biomedical psychiatry means that it increasingly emulates the natural sciences and exists behind a 'scientific patina'.[7] This in turn renders the interrogation of the extent to which normativities inform who is deemed to be 'ill' or 'well'; 'normal', or 'abnormal'—and thus in need of (pharmacological) treatment—more difficult.

To fulfil the book's chief aim, I harness the words of women (self-) diagnosed with SAD, imparted to me through interviews. Themes from their testimonies are placed into dialogue with diagnostic criteria and viewed through a feminist science studies and anti-psychiatry lens. The stories of these women are at the very heart of this work: my theorising about SAD is grounded in their narratives. Moreover, through adopting a position of advocacy, this book prioritises women's own power to define their 'disorder' for themselves. That is, listening to the often-silenced voices of the 'mad'[8] permits the forging of an alternative narrative on women and SAD to that espoused by the psy sciences[9]—disciplines which, in the main, have yet to take heed of women's subjective experiences.

Social Anxiety: A History

Before going any further, it is timely to chart briefly the history of what is now called 'Social Anxiety Disorder'. Literary critic Christopher Lane tells us that the link between shyness and anxiety is not so ahistorical as we might assume.[10] Perhaps the first linkage between them can be found in Robert Burton's seventeenth-century work *The Anatomy of Melancholy,* wherein his citing of Hippocrates describes a man who

> [T]hrough bashfulness, suspicion, and timorousness [...] He dare not come in company, for fear he should be misused, disgraced, overshoot himself in gesture or speeches, or be sick; he thinks every man observes him, aims at him, derides him, owes him malice.[11]

The next notable mention of social anxiety is not to be found until very much later. The psychiatrists—or alienists, as they were then called—of the 1880s 'began viewing shyness as a morbid condition that bordered on pathology'.[12] Specifically, French psychiatrist Paul Hartenberg wrote of 'pathological shyness' in his 1901 work *Les Timides et la Timidité.*[13] Around the same time, French psychologist Pierre Janet coined the term 'Social Phobia' (*Phobies Sociales*).[14] As such, it was not until the 1900s that 'Social Phobia' began to be construed as a mental disorder.[15] This is also the time around which Western psychiatry assumed its current form,[16] with madness being subsumed into medicine.[17] Following on from this, the 1930s witnessed the emergence of 'Social Neurosis', which was characterised by 'shyness', 'a tendency to withdraw from social activities', as well as 'sweating, blushing, inability to speak, and shaking'.[18] SAD was formally conceptualised as a distinct disorder in 1965 by psychiatrists Isaac M. Marks and Michael Graham Gelder who, in their small scale study, described individuals who 'became anxious primarily when required to participate in social situations'. This group exhibited a fear of blushing and would 'shak[e] when the center of attention'.[19]

SAD entered the second edition of the American Psychiatric Association's (APA) *Diagnostic and Statistical Manual of Mental Disorders* (*DSM*) in 1968.[20] The *DSM* will be important going forward in this book, since its most recent iteration, the *DSM-5*, is the psychiatric diagnostic manual used by mental health professionals in the US and worldwide today. It is particularly significant in the US since individuals therein usually require a *DSM-5*-recognised diagnosis in order to be able to claim for the cost of their treatment on their insurance.[21] This means that the manual occupies a pivotal place in both medical, and popular, conceptions of mental distress in the US. In turn, this has influenced conceptions of mental distress in the UK.

The *second* edition of the *DSM* is especially key, for it entailed a shift from conceptualising what were termed 'mental disorders' as *reactions* to 'permanent, even innate conditions':[22] for example, 'schizophrenic reaction' became 'schizophrenia'.[23] Psychiatrist Sami Timimi provides commentary on this newer conceptualisation in the present day:

> When a clinician claims that a patient [...] has ADHD [...] they [are] trying to turn something based on subjective opinion into something that appears empirical [...] they are [...] turning concepts into something that appears as if it exists as a fact in the natural world [...] ADHD is a 'real' disorder that exists in their brains and is potentially lifelong.[24]

In the decade following the release of the *DSM*'s second edition, the SAD diagnosis was not developed a great deal further. The 1980s, however, witnessed the 'transformation of shyness into a disease'.[25] This occurred within the context of the development of the *DSM-III-R*, to which Social Phobia was added as a diagnostic category,[26] and was facilitated 'behind closed doors of carefully vetted committee meetings'[27] by 'a small group of self-selecting'[28]—and 'primarily white, high-status, [and] male'[29]—American psychiatrists.[30] Sociologist Susie Scott contends that since this time, '[T]he diagnostic label has been applied to an increasing number of people who would once have been seen as "just shy".'[31] This reframing of shyness conceptualised it as stemming 'not from psychological conflicts or social tensions, but rather from a chemical imbalance or faulty neurotransmitters in the brain'.[32] This parallels the shift in terminology which occurred with the *DSM*'s second edition, and is a prime example of what Foucault describes as a 'specification of individuals' in his account of the history of the human sciences.[33] That is, Foucault tells us that while homosexuality used to be 'a category of forbidden acts',[34] its classification constructed 'a personage, a past, a case history, and a childhood'.[35] Analogously, the move from describing a mental disorder as a *reaction* to something one *is* renders it 'everywhere present in him: at the root of all his actions because it [is] their insidious and indefinitely active principle [...] It [is] consubstantial with him [...] a singular nature'.[36]

Prior to the *DSM-III-R*'s publication in 1987, SAD had remained somewhat under-researched within the psy sciences, causing psychiatrist Michael R. Liebowitz et al. to term it the 'neglected anxiety disorder' in 1985.[37] The next eight years saw increasing interest in SAD, which led to its being named 'one of the most common psychiatric diagnoses in the Western world'.[38] In 2007, the US National Comorbidity Survey estimated SAD's prevalence in the US population to be 7.1%,[39] with other estimates reaching as high as 18.7%.[40]

As dialogue surrounding SAD grew, so too did speculation on how best to treat it. Dr Murray Stein, who was involved in shyness studies at the University of California, was often present on US television and in pharmaceutical literature alike, wherein he encouraged the public to seek treatment for their social anxiety.[41] The 'Disorder of the Decade' made headlines:[42] the public were told, 'You're Not Shy, You're Sick',[43] and that 'Easing Stage Fright Could Be as Simple as Swallowing a Pill'.[44] Shyness had become subject to 'medicalisation': it had been made medical.[45] Medicalisation entails the transformation of societal problems and human variation into individual problems and pathologies, respectively, and is achieved by the application of diagnostic categories and disease labels. Remedies are then purported to lie in pharmaceutical or behavioural interventions.[46]

Author Lisa Appignanesi uses Columbia University's (now defunct) mental health screening programme, Teen Screen, as a means to critique the medicalisation of mental distress. Teen Screen, she posits, exemplifies the way in which people 'learn the brackets and language into which they can wedge their often inchoate feelings. These are then arranged into today's fashionable diagnoses [...such as] social anxiety disorder, for which Paxil has been widely sold'.[47] Crucially, she points out that Teen Screen may have edged 'the common teenage "social anxiety" into the category of illness'.[48] Feminist psychologist Paula J. Caplan similarly comments on the

> [P]roliferation of television commercials for prescription drugs, many [of which] include a description of an ordinary phenomenon (such as shyness), the relabeling of it (shyness becomes 'Social Anxiety *Disorder*') in ways that alarm people because the message is that they are mentally ill, and finally the announcement that a brand-name drug is just what the 'disordered' person needs.[49]

Feminist activist Sasha Claire McInnes provides a parody of such pharmaceutical advertisements thus:

> Are you shy? Having trouble feeling comfortable with people?
> Don't despair. While you may have long considered shyness to be just another element of your personality, medical 'science' has decided that this trait is the expression of a chronic mental disorder. The American Psychiatric Association asserts that there are 35 million people adrift on a sea of morbid shyness (Social Phobia) and the US Federal Drug Agency (FDA), in May 1992, gave approval to SmithKlineBeecham to market Paxil as the fix.[50]

Although pharmacological treatment is not marketed so aggressively in the UK—we do not (yet!) have direct-to-consumer advertisements—SAD persists today as a distinct mental disorder in psychiatric diagnostic manuals in both countries. The *DSM-5* boasts 'Social Anxiety Disorder (Social Phobia)'[51] and its UK counterpart, the 10*th* edition of the *International Classification of Diseases* (*ICD-10*), lists 'Social Anxiety Disorder'.[52] The two manuals' criteria for psychiatric diagnoses are concurrent to the extent that, beginning with the *DSM-IV*,[53] the APA released an 'International Version' of the manual wherein diagnostic codes are given alongside their *ICD* 'equivalents'.[54] Despite my analysis being focused primarily on the UK, I have engaged with the *DSM* to a greater degree than the *ICD* because I have found the *DSM*'s accounts of its diagnostic categories to be more comprehensive.

The *DSM*-5's diagnostic criteria for SAD are as follows:

A. Marked fear or anxiety about one or more social situations in which the individual is exposed to possible scrutiny by others. Examples include social interactions (e.g., having a conversation, meeting unfamiliar people), being observed (e.g., eating or drinking), and performing in front of others (e.g., giving a speech).
   Note: In children, the anxiety must occur in peer settings and not just during interactions with adults.
B. The individual fears that he or she will act in a way or show anxiety symptoms that will be negatively evaluated (i.e., will be humiliating or embarrassing; will lead to rejection or offend others).
C. The social situations almost always provoke fear or anxiety.

Note: In children, the fear or anxiety may be expressed by crying, tantrums, freezing, clinging, shrinking, or failing to speak in social situations.

D. The social situations are avoided or endured with intense fear or anxiety.
E. The fear or anxiety is out of proportion to the actual threat posed by the social situation and to the sociocultural context.
F. The fear, anxiety, or avoidance is persistent, typically lasting for six months or more.
G. The fear, anxiety, or avoidance causes clinically significant distress or impairment in social, occupational, or other important areas of functioning.
H. The fear, anxiety, or avoidance is not attributable to the physiological effects of a substance (e.g., a drug of abuse, a medication) or another medical condition.
I. The fear, anxiety, or avoidance is not better explained by the symptoms of another mental disorder, such as panic disorder, body dysmorphic disorder, or autism spectrum disorder.
J. If another medical condition (e.g., Parkinson's disease, obesity, disfigurement from burns or injury) is present, the fear, anxiety, or avoidance is clearly unrelated or is excessive.

Specify if:

Performance only: If the fear is restricted to speaking or performing in public.[55]

Why Research Social Anxiety in Women?

Since being dubbed the 'neglected anxiety disorder' in 1985,[56] SAD has been subject to increased research within the psy sciences. Yet, research outside of these disciplines, and particularly concerning women—among whom SAD appears to be more prevalent[57]—is still lacking.[58] As such, critical analysis which interrogates the extent to which women's socialisation contributes to their experiences of social anxiety is long overdue and crucial, especially since psy science explanations for this discrepancy have tended to focus on biologically reductive arguments:[59] that is, hormones, genetics, and reproductive processes are explored as possible causes. Theoretical approaches similar to that which this book adopts have been applied to other psychiatric diagnoses overrepresented in women including Eating Disorders,[60] Depression,[61] and, retrospectively, Hysteria.[62] However, SAD has hitherto not been met with the same scrutiny.

The book's approach is informed by the 'anti-psychiatry' movement, the roots of which we can trace back to the 1960s. Forming as a critique of the emerging field of psychiatry, it sought to render 'mental illnesses' intelligible, or comprehensible, as rational responses to one's circumstances. Indeed, Ronald David Laing, one of the movement's forerunners, famously described insanity as 'a perfectly rational adjustment to an insane world'.[63] While the movement has primarily directed its attentions to schizophrenia and psychosis,[64] this book applies tenets of anti-psychiatry to SAD in women.

The book's conceptual framework is also informed by feminism, specifically feminist science studies. That is, it seeks to expose implicit gender biases in both diagnostic criteria and the way that psychiatry treats women presenting with distress—distress which can often be understood by considering women's subordinated social position. I am inspired by thinkers such as Jane M. Ussher[65] and Phylis Chesler[66] whose research provides a feminist response to anti-psychiatry. Feminist literary critic Elaine Showalter writes on why this response is needed in noting that a number of Laing's case studies feature women who are struggling with resolving conflicting ideas about femininity. Yet, '[T]hese potential theories of gender are not developed in themselves.'[67]

By homing in on women's social anxiety, this book engenders a broader critique of the biological focus which pervades present-day discourses, both inside and outside of psychiatry, on mental distress. It also problematises these discourses' preoccupation with changing the individual: also called the social,[68] or individual, pathology model. That is, '[S]ocially created problems are often the causes of people's pain, but that pain is often mistakenly attributed to factors within the individuals.'[69] Like medicalisation, this directs attention towards the individual and away from (changing) the social structure.[70] Social psychologist Elliott George Mishler speaks to the interplay between medicalisation and the individual pathology model in putting forth that 'medical discourses may frame diseases as a deviation from normal functioning, but in some cases it is appropriate to ask, "deviant for whom?"'.[71]

To explore why social anxiety could be construed as a form of deviance, it is salient to review Scott's exposition of shyness as a type of rule-breaking in interactions. '[I]n everyday life', Scott tells us, '[T]here is an expectation that "normal" (non-shy) people will display a certain level of interactional competence.'[72] The shy person presents 'a threat to this order in that their "moves" are unexpected and uncoordinated with those around them'.[73] Moreover, '[S]hyness in itself can be perceived as such a threat to the flow of interaction, insofar as it is sometimes misinterpreted as rudeness or aloofness.'[74]

We can develop Scott's analysis further in considering that 'women are positioned (and position themselves) as bearing full responsibility for relationships'.[75] By extension, they are held responsible for the feelings, emotions, and even the experiences of others to a far greater extent than men. Their being perceived as a threat to the flow of interaction is thus *doubly* threatening by virtue of their contravention of not only social, but *gendered* norms. Scott argues that, rather than altering normative expectations vis-à-vis interactions, '[i]t is easier and more socially facilitative to blame the individual' and label them[76]—for our purposes, as having Social Anxiety Disorder.

The positioning of the socially anxious woman as disordered and in need of treatment such that she can function in society therefore maintains the very social conditions which—as we shall see when delving into participants' stories—likely contributed to her social anxiety in the first instance. This book's purpose is therefore to refute the individual pathology model as applied to SAD in women by devoting attention to the 'social origins'[77] of this form of mental distress.

A Note on Terminology

Keen-eyed readers will already have noticed my use of quotation marks around such terms as 'mental illness' and 'disorder'. On terminology, Caplan raises a salient point, with which I agree, in noting that 'since language helps shape thought, the precise words we use are important'.[78] The terms I use throughout this book have thus been carefully chosen such that they are congruent with a social approach to mental distress as opposed to a biomedical one. The rationale underpinning this is outlined by social work scholar Jerry Tew:

> The label 'mental illness', and the diagnostic terminologies that go with a biomedical approach, can impact on how people see themselves and are seen by others: it can situate them as passive 'patients' waiting to be cured by experts, and certain aspects of their experience may become invalidated or marginalized.[79]

Therefore, following Tew,

> I have chosen to use the term 'mental distress' to denote experiences that go beyond the upsets, losses and challenges of everyday life. This is a term with which many people who use mental health services are comfortable as it does not imply illness, incapacity or inferiority.[80]

On specific experiences of mental distress, hereafter, 'SAD' and 'Social Anxiety Disorder' (capitalised) will be used when referring to diagnostic categories; 'social anxiety' and 'socially anxious' (lower-case) will be used to describe the unpathologised phenomena: discomfort or unease in interacting with others and fear of being evaluated in a negative light. This distinction is necessary since it provides a means by which I can describe these experiences without endorsing the psychiatric conception of them as illness.

As far as possible, I use de-medicalised language around other characteristics and behaviours that have been pathologised by the psy sciences. I deploy the terms 'sadness' and 'unhappiness', as opposed to 'depression'; eating *problems* as opposed to eating *disorders*; 'nervousness' and 'apprehension' instead of 'anxiety', and so on. My use of capitalised terms is, again, reserved for discussing diagnostic categories.

Interviewing Socially Anxious Women

This book is based on interviews with seven women. Readers may note that my sample size is on the smaller side, but this is by design: it allowed for the collection of incredibly deep and detailed narratives which would not have been possible with a larger sample. Such rich testimonies from women (self-)diagnosed with SAD themselves are notably absent from extant work, and herein lies one of the book's key contributions. Indeed, it is here that I wish to draw on feminist psychologist Sara L. McClelland and colleagues'[81] exposition of a sentiment originally expressed by psychologists Virginia Braun and Victoria Clarke. That is, '[T]he richness of information provided and the theoretical framing of the research project are the most meaningful indicators of robustness, rather than the number of participants.'[82] As such, it is not my intention for my findings to be generalisable to a much wider population, which is often the rationale for using a larger sample. Rather, participants' testimonies are intended to be illustrative of the complexities and gendered character of experiences of SAD.

Participants were recruited by a variety of methods. Some were socially anxious women known to me who were asked if they wished to participate. Others were recruited through research events at my university: when discussing my work, several women volunteered when I revealed that I was still seeking participants! Further participants were recruited via advertisements in my institutional email signature and on my university research page. Additional participants were recruited by referral from friends and colleagues and—using 'snowball sampling'[83]—existing participants.

I interviewed some women in a mutually agreed public place—such as a coffee shop or library—while others preferred to be interviewed by telephone, video call, or email. Each interview was semi-structured, which allowed participants to lead the discussion and describe their experiences 'in their own words'.[84] At the same time, it avoided the potential pitfalls of *un*structured interviews between both a socially anxious interviewer and interviewee—periods of silence, awkwardness, and stunted discussion—by providing a set of five broad questions on which I could fall back.

Each woman was interviewed once with the average duration being an hour and twenty minutes. Interviews were audio recorded, transcribed, and analysed using Braun and Clarke's six steps of general thematic analysis.[85] I also employed member checking:[86] participants were given access to their transcripts as well as my analysis of what they had said. They could then alter their transcripts and check that I had interpreted their narratives as they intended.

Participant Profiles and Intersectionality

Who are the socially anxious women in my sample? Below I introduce each participant and include key characteristics pertinent to the research:[87]

- Farah is a woman of colour in her late thirties and is pursuing a PhD in the arts. After moving from her home country in Western Asia a few years ago, she now lives in the Midlands in the UK with her husband. She spoke about her experiences with Generalised Anxiety Disorder.
- Amy is in her late twenties and is studying for a doctorate in literature. After moving from the US upon completing her undergraduate

degree, she now lives in the Midlands in the UK. She has a heart defect, chronic migraine, and shared her experiences of Depression and Generalised Anxiety Disorder.

- Originally from continental Europe, Daniella moved to the UK to complete her undergraduate degree and is now reading for a PhD in the sciences. She is in her late twenties and lives in the Midlands with her boyfriend. She has lived experience of Anorexia Nervosa, Binge Eating Disorder, and Attention Deficit Hyperactivity Disorder.
- Ellen is a humanities graduate in her late twenties. She works for an NGO in the South of England. She has lived experience of Joint Hypermobility Syndrome, Depression, and Seasonal Affective Disorder.
- Olivia is in her late twenties and is pursuing a PhD in the social sciences. She shared her experience of Depression.
- Phoebe is a social sciences academic based in London and is in her late twenties. She has lived experience of Obsessive Compulsive Disorder and is autistic.
- Ria is a woman of colour who comes from a British-Punjabi family. After completing her master's degree, she now works as a scientist. She lives with her husband in the Midlands and she spoke about her experiences with Bulimia Nervosa and Depression.

Given the intersecting identities of participants, I will consider multiple 'vectors of oppression and privilege'[88] in exploring their experiences. As scholar Kimberlé Crenshaw outlines in her seminal works on intersectionality,[89] using a single axis framework to explore discrimination leaves the experiences of those multiply burdened poorly understood, for 'the intersectional experience is greater than the sum' of the individual axes of oppression.[90]

Readers may notice that participants are all relatively well-educated,[91] and this lent itself well to their giving feedback on my analysis through member checking, thereby affording them greater control over their narratives—with me remaining true to their intended meaning to a greater extent—than would otherwise have been possible. It is also important to point out that although my sample *is* diverse, there are voices from certain groups that are not as well-represented as others. These include youth (16–24) and older women. Another noteworthy area is sexuality: although none of the women mentioned their sexuality in their interviews, all but one mentioned either currently being, or having previously been, in a relationship with a man. While this does not preclude their being under the LGBTQIA+ umbrella, it suggests that my data are most relevant to heterosexual(-passing) women. Taking all of this into account, I echo feminist psychologists Joan C. Chrisler and Ingrid Johnston-Robledo who, at the start of their opus *Women's Embodied Self*, state that

> In many instances in this book there were insufficient data to address diverse women's experiences as thoroughly as we would have liked. Readers are encouraged to think critically about the data that exist and whether they point to generalizable phenomena.[92]

A Note on Inclusion Criteria

Since both femininities[93] and psychiatric diagnoses[94] are culturally constructed and situated, the book's remit is primarily the UK and, to a lesser extent, the US. I engage with UK and US psychiatric diagnostic manuals and participants were required to have lived in the Anglosphere for at least three years.

Participants also needed to be a woman with SAD, either diagnosed by a medical professional or self-diagnosed. My decision to include the self-diagnosed was one of pragmatism. Firstly, one-third of individuals are not told their diagnosis when seeking treatment in primary care—which is where the UK's publicly funded healthcare system, the National Health Service (NHS), recommends first seeking help for SAD[95]—irrespective of presenting complaint.[96] Secondly, healthcare is not universally accessible.[97] Although the philosophy underpinning the NHS is that healthcare is free at the point of delivery and available to all, this is not always the case in practice. Investment in mental health services has been likened to a 'postcode lottery' by mental health charity *Mind*[98] and, against a backdrop of budget cuts in a climate of austerity,[99] mental health services have been badly affected.[100] In addition, the Covid-19 pandemic entailed the shutting down of non-Covid-19 services during the 'first wave', which further reduced availability. This created a backlog[101] which meant waiting times increased even more:[102] the number of patients waiting longer than a year for treatment, including access to mental health services, increased *81-fold* between 2019 and 2020.[103] Ergo, individuals who are in a position to be able to obtain private healthcare are more likely to hold a formal diagnosis. An article from the Royal College of Psychiatrists outlines this rather well in sharing Evangeline's story, 'who ***had to get private treatment*** after waiting months on the NHS':

> My mental health spiralled [...] I saw a mental health specialist at CAMHS but didn't hear anything from them for months [...] *Things got so bad that my family had no option but to book me in for private treatment.*[104]

Evangeline's story leaves me wondering about countless others left by the wayside. What of those whose families do not have the wherewithal to book them in for private treatment? What becomes of individuals whose families are not as supportive as Evangeline's? What about people who do not even *have* families? These individuals do not get treatment *or* diagnosis. As such, in not requiring an official diagnosis, this book provides a platform for a diverse sample of women, with intersecting identities, to tell their stories when they might not otherwise have had the opportunity.

My decision to include self-diagnosed women was also made in light of the observation that psychiatric diagnoses are descriptive[105] as opposed to representing an underlying cause.[106] To insist upon an official diagnosis would risk endorsing the idea that social anxiety is caused by something innate and biological. I thus shaped my inclusion criteria on the basis of my critical conception of psychiatric diagnoses. This involved problematising biological reductionism[107] and drawing on existing critiques of psychiatric diagnoses which describe them as disempowering,[108] stigmatising,[109] and diminishing of personhood.[110]

With that said, diagnoses *can* be empowering:[111] they can be used as a means by which to resist the pathological meaning originally ascribed to the given label. In writing about homosexuality, Foucault calls this phenomenon 'reverse discourse'.[112] Following Foucault, philosopher Ian Hacking tells us that the term 'homosexual' was originally 'applied by the knowers to the known',[113] but was subsequently 'taken up' by those it sought to describe, resulting in gay liberation, gay pride, and coming 'out'. In the spirit of relativising the power of psychiatry, my decision to include women who are self-diagnosed is undergirded by the idea that *psychiatric diagnoses are useful insofar as they serve the individual*, and individuals are free to choose the terms which they feel describe their experience.[114]

Including self-diagnosed women was also inspired by the thoughts of philosophers Ginger A. Hoffman and Jennifer L. Hansen on how 'the self is, fundamentally, constituted by a narrative one tells about oneself'[115] and 'this narrative almost certainly absorbs elements from surrounding cultural scripts'.[116] Since it is these scripts—informed by psychiatric and popular discourses alike—which position socially anxious women as 'mentally ill', these women's experiences of SAD are explorable *with or without an official diagnosis*.

In keeping with this, Ussher speaks to the interplay between these psychiatric and popular discourses in writing that 'we signal our psychic pain, our deep distress, through culturally sanctioned "symptoms", which allows our distress to be positioned as "real"'.[117] She elaborates:

> At the beginning of the 21st century the 'legitimate' symptoms of madness are laid out for all to see in the DSM [*sic*]. As new diagnoses are added with each edition (and others, such as hysteria or homosexuality, removed), details of the necessary symptoms for diagnosis are circulated through interactions with the psy-professions, or through pharmaceutical company advertising, media discussion of madness, and 'self-help' diagnostic websites. Is it surprising that so many women self-diagnose with these disorders and then come forward for professional confirmation of their pathological state?[118]

Indeed, sociologist and anthropologist Paul ten Have has noted the tendency for self-diagnosis to precede official diagnosis, with official diagnosis then being confirmatory.[119] By way of example, at a particularly strained period in my own life, I went to my GP for 'Depression'. During my appointment, I found myself parroting the archetypal symptoms—loss of appetite, tiredness, tearfulness—only realising afterwards that I had given this 'textbook' account because it seemed, and indeed proved to be, the quickest, easiest, and most efficient way to secure the treatment (a change in SSRI) from which I thought I would benefit.

Diagnostic and Treatment Protocols in the UK

As with Depression,[120] the NHS recommends first seeking help for SAD by going to one's GP.[121] The National Institute for Health and Care Excellence (NICE), which writes treatment guidance for the NHS, lists the following as treatment modalities for SAD: Cognitive Behavioural Therapy (CBT), CBT-based supported self-help, pharmacological interventions (chiefly, selective serotonin reuptake inhibitors (SSRIs)), and short-term psychodynamic psychotherapy.[122] The order in which these options are implemented depends on the individual's preferences and their response to treatment,[123] and—as per the point I made earlier—the availability of therapy locally. As we will see in Chap. 4, participants had experienced a combination of these treatments at different times, and this certainly resonates with my own experience: I have tried a number of different SSRI/SNRIs and, on first going to my GP at the age of 20 with the presenting complaint of 'anxiety', I was given the telephone number of a therapy service to call in order to put myself on the waiting list for an appointment. Ironically, one facet of my social anxiety at the time was a particularly severe fear of using the telephone!

Researcher Positionality

My experiences of social anxiety as a woman have undoubtedly influenced my decision to research this topic and ultimately write this book, for it 'means something' to me.[124] Feminist researchers before me have noted that drawing on one's first-hand experience can prove valuable.[125] This is true not only in terms of establishing rapport with participants during interviews,[126] but in terms of my having a privileged episteme from which to theorise about other women's narratives. My approach to this research is also reflexive:[127] I acknowledge my interconnectedness with the participants[128] and how this has shaped the project.

Structure of the Book

This book is formed of seven chapters. The chapter following this one describes my theoretical approach—a blend of feminism and anti-psychiatry—and provides a review of research which informs the book's conceptual framework. This comprises critical scholarship which has been used to problematise other gendered psychiatric diagnoses, such as Female Sexual Dysfunction (FSD) and Pre-menstrual Dysphoric Disorder (PMDD). Chapters 3, 4, 5, and 6 foreground the interviews I conducted with fellow socially anxious women. Therein, I theorise their narratives using my conceptual framework. Chapter 3 deals with help-seeking, as well as 'co-morbidities' and their interplay with normative ideals of femininity. Chapter 4 begins by focussing on participants' experiences of diagnosis and treatment, before forging a holistic understanding of women's SAD. Chapter 5 homes in on participants' fears of negative evaluation, outlining how these concerns are not limited to their bodies, but extend to their whole selves. Chapter 6 develops this further in exploring participants' accounts of cultivating an acceptable outward, or 'false', self which comports with feminine norms and others' expectations. The final chapter draws the book to a close in offering thoughts on where we go from here and some personal reflections.

True to the aims of anti-psychiatry, in what follows I seek to render intelligible the experiences of the women who shared their stories with me. Likewise, in the spirit of feminist analyses of other gendered psychiatric diagnoses, I explore how gendered socialisation shapes the socially anxious woman's experience.

Notes

1. Albert Camus, *The Fall [La Chute]*, trans. Justin O'Brien (Penguin: Harmondsworth, 1957[1956]), p. 59.
2. Thomas S. Szasz, *The Myth of Mental Illness: Foundations of a Theory of Personal Conduct* (New York: Harper and Row, 1974), p. 1.
3. Ibid., throughout.
4. Patricia Fallon, Melanie A. Katzman, and Susan C. Wooley (eds.), *Feminist Perspectives on Eating Disorders* (New York: Guilford Press, 1996).
   Susie Orbach, *Fat Is a Feminist Issue* (London: Arrow Books Limited, 1986).
   Susie Orbach, *Bodies* (New York: Picador, 2009).
   Susie Orbach, *Hunger Strike: Starving amidst Plenty* (London and New York: Karnac, 2005).
5. Janet Stoppard, *Understanding Depression: Feminist Social Constructionist Approaches* (London: Routledge, 2014).
6. Not to be confused with the diagnosis 'Seasonal Affective Disorder'.
7. Carl I. Cohen, 'The Biomedicalization of Psychiatry: A Critical Overview', *Community Mental Health Journal*, 29.6 (1993), 509–21 https://doi.org/10.1007/BF00754260 p. 517.
8. Michel Foucault, *History of Madness*, ed. Jean Khalfa, trans. Jonathan Murphy and Jean Khalfa (London and New York: Routledge, 2006) [*Folie et Déraison: Histoire de la Folie à L'âge Classique*, 1961]).
   Readers should note that 'mad' is not used here in a pejorative manner, for the term has been reclaimed. For instance, there now exists a Mad Pride Movement as well as a burgeoning field of Mad Studies. For more on Mad Pride, see Summer Schrader, Nev Jones, and Mona Shattell, 'Mad Pride: Reflections on Sociopolitical Identity and Mental Diversity in the Context of Culturally Competent Psychiatric Care', *Issues in Mental Health Nursing* (2013), 34.1, 62–64 https://doi.org/10.3109/01612840.2012.740769

For more on Mad Studies, see Brenda A. LeFrançois, Robert Menzies, and Geoffrey Reaume (eds). *Mad Matters: A Critical Reader in Canadian Mad Studies* (Toronto: Canadian Scholars' Press, 2013).

9. For more on alternative narratives on women's SAD, see Katie Masters, 'Women's Experiences of Social Anxiety Disorder: Privileging Marginalised Perspectives and Rewriting Dominant Narratives', *International Mad Studies Journal*, 1.1 (2022), e1–21 https://doi.org/10.58544/imsj.v1i1.5244
10. Christopher Lane, *Shyness: How Normal Behavior Became a Sickness* (Yale University Press, 2007) https://ebookcentral.proquest.com/lib/bham/reader.action?docID=3420940 [accessed 6 January 2021] p. 11.
11. Hippocrates, quoted in Robert Burton, *The Anatomy of Melancholy: What it Is, with all the Kinds, Causes, Symptoms, Prognostics, and Several Cures of It* (London: William Tegg, 1854[1621]), p. 253.
12. Lane, *Shyness*, p. 14.
13. Paul Hartenberg, *Les Timides et la Timidité* (Paris: Félix Alcan, 1901).
14. Pierre Janet, *Les Obsessions et la Psychasthénie* (Paris: Félix Alcan, 1903), 2 Vols., 1:210.
15. Thierry Haustgen, 'À Propos du Centenaire de la Psychasthénie (1903): Les Troubles Obsessionnels-Compulsifs dans la Psychiatrie Française: Revue Historique', *Annales Médico-psychologiques, Revue Psychiatrique*, 162.6 (2004), 427–40 https://doi.org/10.1016/j.amp.2003.09.012
16. Joel Kovel, 'The American Mental Health Industry', in *Critical Psychiatry*, ed. by David Ingleby (New York: Pantheon, 1980), 72–101.
17. Michel Foucault, *Madness and Civilization: A History of Insanity in the Age of Reason* [based on an abridged version of *Folie et Déraison: Histoire de la Folie à L'âge Classique*], trans. Richard Howard (London and New York: Routledge, 2001[1961]).
18. Paul Schilder, 'The Social Neurosis', *Psychoanalytic Review*, 25 (1938), 1–19 https://psycnet.apa.org/record/1938-02478-001 [accessed 3 January 2021] p. 1.
19. Isaac M. Marks and Michael Graham Gelder, 'Different Ages of Onset in Varieties of Phobia', *American Journal of Psychiatry*, 123.2 (1966), 218–21 https://doi.org/10.1176/ajp.123.2.218 p. 218.
20. American Psychiatric Association [APA], *Diagnostic and Statistical Manual of Mental Disorders*, 2nd edn [*DSM-II*] (Washington, DC: American Psychiatric Association Publishing, 1968).
21. For more on how this works, and how the codes are related to *ICD* codes, see APA, *Insurance Implications of DSM-5* (2013) https://www.psychiatry.org/File%20Library/Psychiatrists/Practice/DSM/APA_DSM_Insurance-Implications-of-DSM-5.pdf [accessed 27 June 2023].
22. Lane, *Shyness*, p. 38.
23. Ibid.

24. Sami Timimi, 'No More Psychiatric Labels: Why Formal Psychiatric Diagnostic Systems Should Be Abolished', *International Journal of Clinical and Health Psychology*, 14.3 (2014), 208–15 https://doi.org/10.1016/j.ijchp.2014.03.004 p. 210.
25. Lane, *Shyness*, p. 2.
26. Ibid., pp. 2–3.
27. Ibid., p. 2.
28. Ibid.
29. Paula J. Caplan and Lisa Cosgrove, 'Is this Really Necessary?' in *Bias in Psychiatric Diagnosis*, ed. by Paula J. Caplan and Lisa Cosgrove (Northvale: Jason Aronson Inc., 2004), xix–xxxii, p. xx.
30. Lane, *Shyness*, p. 2.
31. Susie Scott, 'The Medicalisation of Shyness: From Social Misfits to Social Fitness', *Sociology of Health and Illness*, 28.2 (2006), 133–53 https://doi.org/10.1111/j.1467-9566.2006.00485.x p. 135.
32. Lane, *Shyness*, p. 2.
33. Michel Foucault, *The Will to Knowledge, The History of Sexuality: I*, trans. Robert Hurley (Harmondsworth: Penguin, 1998), pp. 42–43.
34. Ibid.
35. Ibid.
36. Ibid.
37. Michael R. Liebowitz, Jack M. Gorman, Abby J. Fyer, and Donald F. Klein, 'Social Phobia: Review of a Neglected Anxiety Disorder', *Archives of General Psychiatry*, 42.7 (1985), 729–36 https://doi.org/10.1001/archpsyc.1985.01790300097013
38. Lane, *Shyness*, p. 6.
39. Harvard Medical School, *National Comorbidity Survey* (2007) https://www.hcp.med.harvard.edu/ncs/index.php [accessed 27 June 2023]. See table 2: 12-month prevalence *DSM-IV/WMH-CIDI* disorders by sex and cohort (n = 9282).
40. The figure has been found to vary from 1.9 to 18.7%, depending on where the diagnostic threshold is set. When the threshold is set in accordance with the *DSM-III-R*'s criteria, the figure is given as 7.1%. See Murray B. Stein, John R. Walker, and David R. Forde, 'Setting Diagnostic Thresholds for Social Phobia', *American Journal of Psychiatry*, 151.3 (1994), 408–12 https://doi.org/10.1176/ajp.151.3.408 p. 408.
41. Lane, *Shyness*, pp. 4–5.
42. Psychology Today, *Disorder of the Decade* (1993), https://www.psychologytoday.com/intl/articles/199307/disorder-the-decade [accessed 7 January 2021].
43. Colby Cosh, 'You're not Shy, You're Sick: Psychiatrists Discover a Crippling "Social Anxiety Disorder" that Affects 13% of Us', *The Report* (June 19, 2000), 49–50, cited in Lane, *Shyness*, pp. 4–5.

44. Elyse Tanouye, 'Easing Stage Fright Could Be as Simple as Swallowing a Pill', *Wall Street Journal* (June 30, 1997; Eastern ed.) https://www.wsj.com/articles/SB867615759865100000 [accessed 14 June 2023].
45. Peter Conrad, 'Medicalization and Social Control', *Annual Review of Sociology*, 18 (1992), 209–32 www.jstor.org/stable/2083452 [accessed 3 January 2021].
46. Peter Conrad, *The Medicalization of Society: On the Transformation of Human Conditions into Treatable Disorders* (Baltimore, MD: Johns Hopkins University Press, 2008).
47. Lisa Appignanesi, *Mad, Bad and Sad: A History of Women and the Mind Doctors from 1800 to the Present* (London: Virago, 2008), pp. 531–32.
48. Ibid.
49. Caplan and Cosgrove, 'Is this Really Necessary?', p. xxiv.
50. Sasha Claire McInnes, 'The Political Is Personal–Or, Why Have a Revolution (from within or without) when You Can Have Soma?' *Feminist Review*, 68.1 (2001), 160–66 https://doi.org/10.1080/01417780110042455 p. 160.
51. APA, *Diagnostic and Statistical Manual of Mental Disorders* [*DSM-5*] (Washington, DC: American Psychiatric Association Publishing, 2013) https://ebookcentral.proquest.com/lib/bham/reader.action?docID=1811753 [accessed 6 January 2021].
52. World Health Organization [WHO], 'Social Phobias', *International Classification of Diseases*, 10th edn [*ICD-10*] (2016) https://icd.who.int/browse10/2016/en#/F40.1 [accessed 25 September 2020].
53. Gavin Andrews, Tim Slade, and Lorna Peters, 'Classification in Psychiatry: ICD-10 versus DSM-IV', *The British Journal of Psychiatry*, 174.1 (1999), 3–5 https://doi.org/10.1192/bjp.174.1.3 p. 3.
54. Ibid.
55. APA, *DSM-5*, pp. 202–03.
56. Liebowitz et al., 'Social Phobia'.
57. Several studies report this finding:
    David J. De Wit, Michelle Chandler-Coutts, David R. Offord, Gillian King, Janette McDougall, Jacqueline Specht, and Shannon Stewart, 'Gender Differences in the Effects of Family Adversity on the Risk of Onset of DSM-III-R Social Phobia', *Journal of Anxiety Disorders*, 19.5 (2005), 479–502 https://doi.org/10.1016/j.janxdis.2004.04.010
    Hans-Ulrich Wittchen, Murray B. Stein, and Ronald C. Kessler, 'Social Fears and Social Phobia in a Community Sample of Adolescents and Young Adults: Prevalence, Risk Factors and Co-morbidity', *Psychological Medicine*, 29.2 (1999), 309–23 https://doi.org/10.1017/s0033291798008174

Maya Asher, Anu Asnaani, and Idan M. Aderka, 'Gender Differences in Social Anxiety Disorder: A Review', *Clinical Psychology Review*, 56 (2017), 1–12 https://doi.org/10.1016/j.cpr.2017.05.004

58. Indeed, this gender asymmetry underpins the decision to focus on women in this book and it will be explored further in subsequent chapters.
59. E.g. Margaret Altemus, 'Sex Differences in Depression and Anxiety Disorders: Potential Biological Determinants', *Hormones and Behavior*, 50. 4 (2006), 534–38 https://doi.org/0.1016/j.yhbeh.2006.06.031
    Lisa S. Weinstock, 'Gender Differences in the Presentation and Management of Social Anxiety Disorder', *The Journal of Clinical Psychiatry*, 60 (Suppl9) (1999), 9–13 https://psycnet.apa.org/record/1999-05175-002 [accessed 4 January 2021].
60. Fallon et al., *Feminist Perspectives on Eating Disorders*.
61. Stoppard, *Understanding Depression*.
62. Elaine Showalter, *The Female Malady: Women, Madness, and English Culture* (New York: Pantheon, 1985).
63. Ronald David Laing, quoted in Larry Chang, *Wisdom for the Soul: Five Millennia of Prescriptions for Spiritual Healing* (Washington DC: Gnosophia Publishing, 2006), p. 412.
64. Ronald David Laing, *The Divided Self: An Existential Study in Sanity and Madness* (London: Tavistock Publications Ltd., 1965).
    David Cooper, *Psychiatry and Anti-psychiatry*, 2nd edn (St. Albans: Paladin, 1972).
65. Jane M. Ussher, *Women's Madness: Misogyny or Mental Illness?* (London: Harvester Wheatsheaf, 1991).
66. Phyllis Chesler, *Women and Madness* (London: Allen Lane, 1974).
67. Showalter, *The Female Malady*, p. 231.
68. Milena Büchs, 'Social Pathology', *The Blackwell Encyclopedia of Sociology* (2007) https://doi.org/10.1002/9781405165518.wbeoss173
69. Paula J. Caplan, *When Jonny and Jane Come Marching Home: How all of Us Can Help Veterans* (Hanover, NH: Scribl, 2019), p. iv.
70. Conrad, *The Medicalization of Society*, note 50, p. 152.
71. Elliott George Mishler, 'Critical Perspectives on the Biomedical Model', in *Perspectives in Medical Sociology*, ed. by Phil Brown (Belmont, CA: Wadsworth, 1989) cited in Scott, 'The Medicalisation of Shyness', p. 139.
72. Susie Scott, 'The Shell, the Stranger and the Competent Other: Towards a Sociology of Shyness', *Sociology*, 38.1 (2004), 121–37 https://doi.org/10.1177/0038038504039364 p. 128.
73. Ibid.
74. Susie Scott, 'The Red, Shaking Fool: Dramaturgical Dilemmas in Shyness', *Symbolic Interaction*, 28.1 (2005), 91–110 https://doi.org/10.1525/si.2005.28.1.91 p. 92.

75. Dana Crowley Jack, *Silencing the Self: Women and Depression* (Cambridge, MA: Harvard University Press, 1991).
Helen O'Grady, *Woman's Relationship with Herself: Gender, Foucault, Therapy* (London: Routledge, 2005).
All cited in Jane M. Ussher and Janette Perz, 'PMS as a Gendered Illness Linked to the Construction and Relational Experience of Hetero-Femininity', *Sex Roles*, 68. 1–2 (2013), 132–50 https://doi.org/10.1007/s11199-011-9977-5 p. 136.
76. Scott, 'The Shell, the Stranger and the Competent Other', p. 128.
77. Joan Busfield, *Men, Women and Madness* (Basingstoke: Macmillan, 1996), p. 144.
78. Caplan, *When Jonny and Jane Come Marching Home*, p. 14.
79. Jerry Tew, *Social Approaches to Mental Distress* (Basingstoke: Palgrave Macmillan, 2011), p. 4.
80. Ibid., p. 5.
81. Sara L. McClelland, Jennifer D. Rubin, and Jose A. Bauermeister, 'Adapting to Injustice: Young Bisexual Women's Interpretations of Microaggressions', *Psychology of Women Quarterly*, 40.4 (2016), 532–50 https://doi.org/10.1177/0361684316664514 p. 536.
82. Virginia Braun and Victoria Clarke, *Successful Qualitative Research: A Practical Guide for Beginners* (London, England: Sage, 2013).
83. Lucy Gibson, '"Type Me Your Answer." Generating Interview Data via Email', in *Collecting Qualitative Data: A Practical Guide to Textual and Virtual Techniques*, ed. by Virginia Braun, Victoria Clarke and Debra Gray (Cambridge, UK and New York, NY: Cambridge University Press, 2017), 213–34, p. 223.
84. Hilary Arksey and Peter T. Knight, *Interviewing for Social Scientists: An Introductory Resource with Examples* (London and Thousand Oaks, California: Sage Publications, 1999), p. 82.
85. Braun and Clarke, 'Using Thematic Analysis in Psychology'.
86. Linda Birt, Suzanne Scott, Debbie Cavers, Christine Campbell, and Fiona Walter, 'Member Checking: A Tool To Enhance Trustworthiness or Merely a Nod to Validation?', *Qualitative Health Research*, 26.13 (2016), 1802–11 https://doi.org/10.1177/1049732316654870
87. Names and any identifying characteristics have been altered for the sake of participant anonymity.
88. George Ritzer, *Contemporary Sociological Theory and Its Classical Roots: The Basics* (Boston: McGraw-Hill, 2007), p. 204.
89. Kimberlé Crenshaw, 'Demarginalizing the Intersection of Race and Sex: A Black Feminist Critique of Antidiscrimination Doctrine, Feminist Theory and Antiracist Politics', *University of Chicago Legal Forum*, 1.8 (1989), 139–67 http://chicagounbound.uchicago.edu/uclf/vol1989/iss1/8 [accessed 27 June 2023].

Kimberlé Crenshaw, 'Mapping the Margins: Intersectionality, Identity Politics, and Violence against Women of Color', *Stanford Law Review*, 43.6 (1991), 1241–99 https://doi.org/10.2307/1229039

90. Crenshaw, 'Demarginalizing the Intersection of Race and Sex', p. 140.
91. In a UK context, which is from where participants were all drawn, readers should note that well-educated does not inevitably mean upper or middle class, as might be the case in a US context. In the UK, many working-class people go to university.
92. Joan C. Chrisler and Ingrid Johnston-Robledo, 'Woman's Embodied Self: An Introduction', in *Woman's Disembodied Self: Feminist Perspectives on Identity and Image*, ed. by Joan C. Chrisler and Ingrid Johnston-Robledo, (Washington, D.C.: American Psychological Association, 2018), 3–14, p. 6.
93. Showalter, *The Female Malady.*
94. Laurence J. Kirmayer, 'Cultural Psychiatry in Historical Perspective', in *Textbook of Cultural Psychiatry*, ed. by Kamaldeep Bhui and Dinesh Bhugra (Cambridge: Cambridge University Press, 2007), 3–19.
95. NHS, *Social Anxiety Disorder (Social Phobia)* (2020) https://www.nhs.uk/conditions/social-anxiety/ [accessed 7 January 2021].
96. John Heritage, 'Revisiting Authority', in *Diagnosis as Cultural Practice*, ed. by Judith Felson Duchan and Dana Kovarsky (Mouton de Gruyter, 2005) https://r2.vlereader.com/Reader?ean=9783110199802 [accessed 6 January 2021] 83–102, p. 88.
97. Jennifer Vanderminden and Jennifer J. Esala, 'Beyond Symptoms: Race and Gender Predict Anxiety Disorder Diagnosis', *Society and Mental Health*, 9.1 (2019), 111–25 https://doi.org/10.1177/2156869318811435 p. 113.

    Sian Ferguson, 'Self-Diagnosing Mental Illness Isn't Perfect, but here's why It Can Be Necessary', *Everyday Feminism* (2017) https://everydayfeminism.com/2017/02/self-diagnosing-mental-illness/ [accessed 7 January 2021].
98. Mind, *NHS Figures Reveal Mental Health Spending Postcode Lottery* (2019) https://www.mind.org.uk/news-campaigns/news/nhs-figures-reveal-mental-health-spending-postcode-lottery/ [accessed 19 February 2021].
99. British Medical Association, *Prioritising Prevention for Population Health* (2019) https://www.bma.org.uk/collective-voice/policy-and-research/public-and-population-health/prioritising-prevention-for-population-health [accessed 7 January 2021].
100. Trade Union Congress, *Breaking Point: The Crisis in Mental Health Funding* (2018) https://www.tuc.org.uk/sites/default/files/Mentalhealthfundingreport2_0.pdf [accessed 10 June 2019].

101. British Medical Association [BMA], *Pressure Points in the NHS* (2021) https://www.bma.org.uk/advice-and-support/nhs-delivery-and-workforce/pressures/pressure-points-in-the-nhs [accessed 22 February 2021].
102. NHS England, *Consultant-led Referral to Treatment Waiting Times Data 2020-21* (2020) https://www.england.nhs.uk/statistics/statistical-work-areas/rtt-waiting-times/rtt-data-2020-21/ [accessed 22 February 2021] cited in Shaun Griffin, 'Covid-19: Waiting Times in England Reach Record Highs', *British Medical Journal* (2020) 370.m3557, 1 https://doi.org/10.1136/bmj.m3557
103. NHS England, *Consultant-led Referral to Treatment Waiting Times.*
104. Royal College of Psychiatrists, *Two-fifths of Patients Waiting for Mental Health Treatment Forced To Resort To Emergency or Crisis Services* (2020) https://www.rcpsych.ac.uk/news-and-features/latest-news/detail/2020/10/06/two-fifths-of-patients-waiting-for-mental-health-treatment-forced-to-resort-to-emergency-or-crisis-services [accessed 23 February 2021]. My emphases.
105. Stijn Vanheule, *Diagnosis and the DSM: A Critical Review* (Basingstoke and New York: Palgrave Macmillan, 2014).
Kenneth S. Kendler and Josef Parnas (eds.), *Philosophical Issues in Psychiatry: Explanation, Phenomenology, and Nosology* (Johns Hopkins University Press, 2008) http://ebookcentral.proquest.com/lib/bham/detail.action?docID=4398485 [accessed 6 January 2021] p. 373.
Alison Faulkner and Vicky Nicholls, *Towards a Radically Different Mental Health System* (n.d.) www.critpsynet.freeuk.com/Faulkner.htm [accessed 7 January 2021].
106. Robert West, Lee Kennedy, and Anna Carr, *The Rehabilitation of Speech, A Textbook of Diagnostic and Corrective Procedures Based upon a Critical Study of Speech Disorders* (Revised edn.) (New York: Harper, 1947), p. 61, cited in Judith Felson Duchan, 'The Diagnostic Practices of Speech-Language Pathologists in America over the Last Century', in Duchan and Kovarsky, *Diagnosis as Cultural Practice*, 201–22, pp. 208–09.
107. Philip Thomas and Patrick Bracken, 'Power, Freedom, and Mental Health: A Postpsychiatry Perspective', in *Liberatory Psychiatry*, ed. by Carl I. Cohen and Sami Timimi (Cambridge: Cambridge University Press, 2008), 35–54, p. 49.
108. David C. Giles and Julie Newbold, 'Self- and Other-diagnosis in User-led Mental Health Online Communities', *Qualitative Health Research*, 21.3 (2010), 419–28 https://doi.org/10.1177/1049732310381388 p. 427.
109. Joseph L. Baird, Stephen P. Hinshaw, and Sheree L. Toth, *The Mark of Shame: Stigma of Mental Illness and an Agenda for Change* (Oxford University Press Incorporated, 2006) http://ebookcentral.proquest.com/lib/bham/detail.action?docID=415914 [accessed 6 January 2021] p. 232.

Ramotse Saunders, Amjad Hindi, and Ipsit Vahia, 'A New Psychiatry for a New World: Postcolonialism, Postmodernism, and the Integration of Premodern Thought into Psychiatry', in *Liberatory Psychiatry*, 205–34, p. 212.

110. Barbara G. Bokhour, 'A Diagnosed Life in an Institutional Setting: Can the Dancer Walk?' in Duchan and Kovarsky, *Diagnosis as Cultural Practice*, 33–63, p. 34.
Judith Felson Duchan and Dana Kovarsky, 'Introduction', in Duchan and Kovarsky, *Diagnosis as Cultural Practice*, 1–14, p. 9.
111. Baird et al., *The Mark of Shame*, p. 232.
112. Foucault, *The Will to Knowledge*, p. 101.
113. Ian Hacking, 'The Looping Effects of Human Kinds', in *Causal Cognition: A Multidisciplinary Debate*, ed. by Dan Sperber, David Premack, and Ann James Premack (Oxford: Oxford University Press, 1995), 351–83 https://doi.org/10.1093/acprof:oso/9780198524021.003.0012 p. 381.
114. Disability Visibility Project, *Abolition Must Include Psychiatry* (2020) https://disabilityvisibilityproject.com/2020/07/22/abolition-must-include-psychiatry/ [accessed 7 January 2021].
115. Daniel C. Dennett, 'The Origins of Selves', *Cogito*, 1 (1989), 163–73 https://doi.org/10.5840/cogito19893348
Owen Flanagan Jr., 'Multiple Identity, Character Transformation, and Self-reclamation', in G. Lynn Stephens and George Graham (eds.), *Philosophical Psychopathology* (Cambridge, MA: MIT Press, 1994).
Marya Schechtman, *The Constitution of Selves* (Ithaca, NY: Cornell University Press, 1996).
Şerife Tekin, 'Self-concept through the Diagnostic Looking Glass: Narratives and Mental Disorder', *Philosophical Psychology*, 24.3 (2011), 357–80 https://doi.org/10.1080/09515089.2011.559622
All cited in Ginger A. Hoffman and Jennifer L. Hansen, 'Prozac or Prosaic Diaries?: The Gendering of Psychiatric Disability in Depression Memoirs', *Philosophy, Psychiatry, and Psychology*, 24.4 (2017), 285–98 https://doi.org/10.1353/ppp.2017.0041 p. 285.
116. Françoise Baylis, 'The Self in Situ: A Relational Account of Personal Identity', in Jocelyn Downie and Jennifer J. Llewellyn (eds.), *Being Relational: Reflections on Relational Theory and Health Law* (Vancouver: UBC Press, 2011).
Hilde Lindemann Nelson, *Damaged Identities, Narrative Repair* (Ithaca, NY: Cornell University Press, 2001).
Tekin, 'Self-concept through the Diagnostic Looking Glass'.
Şerife Tekin, 'How Does the Self Adjudicate Narratives?' *Philosophy, Psychiatry, and Psychology*, 20.1 (2013), 25–28 https://doi.org/10.1353/ppp.2013.0005

Şerife Tekin, 'Self-insight in the Time of Mood Disorders: After the Diagnosis, Beyond the Treatment', *Philosophy, Psychiatry, and Psychology*, 21 (2014), 135–37 https://doi.org/10.1353/ppp.2014.0019

All cited in Hoffman and Hansen, 'Prozac or Prosaic Diaries?', p. 285.

117. Jane M. Ussher, 'Diagnosing Difficult Women and Pathologising Femininity: Gender Bias in Psychiatric Nosology', *Feminism and Psychology*, 23.1 (2013), 63–69 https://doi.org/10.1177/0959353512467968 p. 64
118. Ibid.
119. Paul ten Have, 'Lay Diagnosis in Interaction', *Text and Talk*, 21.1–2 (2008), 251–60 https://doi.org/10.1515/text.1.21.1-2.251 p. 252, cited in Cindy Suopis and Donal Carbaugh, 'Speaking about Menopause: Possibilities for a Cultural Discourse Analysis', in Duchan and Kovarsky, *Diagnosis as Cultural Practice*, 263–76, p. 267.
120. NHS, *Overview – Depression in Adults* (2023) https://www.nhs.uk/mental-health/conditions/depression-in-adults/overview/ [accessed 5 October 2023].
121. NHS, *Social Anxiety Disorder*.
122. NICE, *Interventions for Adults with Social Anxiety Disorder* (2013) https://www.nice.org.uk/guidance/cg159/chapter/1-Recommendations#interventions-for-adults-with-social-anxiety-disorder-2 [accessed 25 September 2020].
123. See NICE, *Interventions for Adults with Social Anxiety Disorder* for the algorithm as to which treatments, and in which order, are prescribed.
124. Ann Oakley, 'Interviewing Women: A Contradiction in Terms', in *Doing Feminist Research*, ed. by Helen Roberts (London: Routledge and Kegan Paul, 1981), 30–61.

Pamela Cotterill and Gayle Letherby, '"Weaving Stories": Personal Auto/biographies in Feminist Research', *Sociology*, 27.1 (1993), 67–80 https://doi.org/10.1177/003803859302700107

Pamela Cotterill and Gayle Letherby, 'The "Person" in the Researcher', in *Studies in Qualitative Methodology, Vol. 4*, ed. by Robert G. Burgess, (London: JAI Press, 1994), 107–36.

Liz Stanley and Sue Wise, *Breaking Out Again: Feminist Ontology and Epistemology* (London: Routledge, 1993).

Jane Ribbens and Rosalind Edwards, *Feminist Dilemmas in Qualitative Research: Public Knowledge and Private Lives* (London: Sage, 1998).

All cited in Gayle Letherby, 'Dangerous Liaisons: An Auto/biography in Research and Research Writing', in *Danger in the Field: Risk and Ethics in Social Research*, ed. by Geraldine Lee-Treweek and Stephanie Linkogle (Taylor and Francis Group, 2000), 91–113 https://ebookcentral.proquest.com/lib/bham/reader.action?docID=166040 [accessed 6 January 2021] p. 95.

125. Oakley, 'Interviewing Women'.
Cotterill and Letherby, '"Weaving Stories"'.
Cotterill and Letherby, 'The "Person" in the Researcher'.
Stanley and Wise, *Breaking Out Again*.
Ribbens and Edwards, *Feminist Dilemmas in Qualitative Research*.
All cited in Letherby, 'Dangerous Liaisons', p. 95.
Elizabeth Mollard, 'Exploring Paradigms in Postpartum Depression Research: The Need for Feminist Pragmatism', *Health Care for Women International*, 36.4 (2015), 378–91 https://doi.org/10.1080/07399332.2014.903951 p. 382.
126. Letherby, 'Dangerous Liaisons', p. 97.
127. Gouldner, *The Coming Crisis*.
128. Mollard, 'Exploring Paradigms in Postpartum Depression Research', pp. 380–81.

CHAPTER 2

Gender, Psychiatry, and Social Anxiety

A proper critical enquiry into the diagnosis 'Social Anxiety Disorder' requires laying some groundwork. To do so, we must journey back not only to see how social anxiety came to be viewed as a psychiatric disorder, but hark back hundreds of years to understand how the medical speciality of psychiatry itself was established. From here, we can chart the biomedical bent that psychiatry's trajectory has tended to assume and the synchronous rising importance of pharmaceutical remedies. In so doing, the interdependency between culture and psychiatric diagnoses is brought to light. A crucial facet of this reciprocity is how certain diagnoses are imbued with norms of femininity. As such, the second portion of this chapter sees a delving into literatures which have drawn on feminist and anti-psychiatry perspectives to critique overtly gendered psychiatric diagnostic categories—Pre-menstrual Dysphoric Disorder (PMDD) and Female Sexual Dysfunction (FSD), to name but a few. In homing in on key tenets therein, I outline how this book's approach to women's SAD will borrow from, and build upon, this extant body of work.

A History of (Anti-)psychiatry

It is usually taken for granted that what we call 'madness' has always been understood in medical terms, but this was not the case until around the nineteenth century.[1] In pre-modern times, Michel Foucault tells us,

K. Masters, *Feminist and Anti-Psychiatry Perspectives on 'Social Anxiety Disorder'*,
https://doi.org/10.1007/978-3-031-48707-1_2

madness was accepted as a different way of existing in the world: a mediator between order and chaos. Foucault likens sanity and madness to 'two threads' which were once 'intertwined',[2] however came to be separated by an 'act of scission'.[3] This led to their being regarded as opposites: to be sane was to be healthful and normal; to be mad was to be unwell and abnormal.

Before madness became medicalised in the nineteenth century, doctors had only a minor role in treating the mad, the duty of care for whom rested with religion and common morality. Foucault explains that the mad began to be institutionalised in the mid-seventeenth century,[4] and this extended into the eighteenth century. Madhouses were also home to the ill, those without work, and the destitute[5]—those who posed a threat to social or financial stability. Since the institutionalisation of the mad involved the congregation of large numbers of mental patients in one place, it established their status as objects of research and facilitated their being classified in much the same way as patients suffering from other diseases.[6] This marked the beginning of madness being studied as a medical phenomenon.

While the early nineteenth century saw the seeds of psychiatry's inclusion in medicine being sown, madness was still not treated as something medical at that time. Moral figures, such as doctor Phillipe Pinel—notable for his 'spectacular unchaining of the mad at Bicêtre'[7]—and Quaker William Tuke were entrusted with treating the mad, and Foucault contends that both men's treatments featured a shift from physical confinement towards mental subjection. This shift is echoed by anti-psychiatrist R. D. Laing's account of psychiatric patients in the twentieth century: he puts forth that, whereas confinement was previously physical, using locked doors, restraints, and straitjackets, newer methods such as 'lobotomies and tranquillizers [...] place the bars of Bedlam and the locked doors *inside* the patient'.[8]

Pinel viewed the mad as being ill, as did other prominent figures of the time, such as psychiatrist Wilhelm Griesinger. Believing madness to be caused by brain lesions, Griesinger hoped that science could provide a cure, and that the stigma-ridden label of 'mad' would be replaced by that of a medical condition.[9] A number of 'cures' were practised in asylums throughout the nineteenth century, including bloodletting and cold water therapy.[10] Female genital mutilation was also practised, with clitoridectomy being endorsed by Isaac Baker Brown in his work *On the Curability of Certain Forms of Insanity, Epilepsy, Catalepsy and Hysteria in Females.*[11]

Indeed, women's sensitivity to mental illness[12] was often blamed on their reproductive systems and linked to pregnancy, menstruation, and menopause.[13] This is exemplified by the innately female disease of Hysteria, which was thought to be caused by a 'wandering womb'. An idea likely originating with Hippocrates,[14] the womb's supposed movement around the body purportedly gave rise to a number of diseases including paralysis and palpitations.[15] Despite Greek physicians Galen's and Soranus of Ephesus's insistence that the uterus cannot move,[16] its alleged mobility remained linked to illness until the modern era.[17] A contemporary example of the inherently feminine being implicated in psychiatric disorder is given by psychologists Jane M. Ussher and Janette Perz in discussing Premenstrual Dysphoric Disorder (PMDD). They characterise this as

> [A]n archetypal example of normal female experience being positioned as mad, resulting in women taking up (or being given) a psychiatric diagnosis, with consequences for how their behaviour is subsequently judged. PMDD sits in the *Diagnostic and Statistical Manual of the American Psychiatric Association*, DSM-4 [*sic*],[18] officially categorising premenstrual mood or behaviour change as pathology.[19]

While the nineteenth century saw the inherently feminine being pathologised, it also saw a fall in the number of women who ran asylums,[20] likely because medicine was deemed to be an inappropriate vocation for women.[21] Early in the nineteenth century, *men* comprised the majority of patients in asylums,[22] but this trend had reversed by the end of the century.[23] Most marked between 1870 and 1910, this shift coincided with middle-class women's organising.[24] Elaine Showalter explains: 'During an era when patriarchal culture felt itself to be under attack by its rebellious daughters, one obvious defence was to label women campaigning for access to the universities, the professions, and the vote as mentally disturbed.'[25] Consequently, 'Victorian psychiatry thus established lunatic asylums increasingly populated by women but supervised by men',[26] and the power to specify what constituted madness lay with the male psychiatrist.[27]

Within these asylums, the nineteenth and early twentieth centuries witnessed the proliferation of more controversial methods. These included insulin therapy; electroconvulsive therapy, which continued into the late 1930s; and lobotomies, with Egas Moniz being awarded a Nobel Prize in 1949 for his performing a frontal leucotomy.[28] Hence, criticism of the asylum, and its ineffective and inhumane methods, started to grow. The pressure group The Mental Hygiene Movement, which sought to improve treatment and conditions in asylums, formed between 1905 and 1910.[29] The view that asylums were 'monuments of therapeutic failure'[30] gained traction, pushing psychiatry instead to establish itself in mental hygiene clinics, centres for child guidance, research centres, and outpatient clinics.[31] Indeed, at the time of writing, those seeking help for SAD are typically treated on an outpatient basis.[32]

The early twentieth century also saw a move from 'home remedies and patent medicines' to professional healthcare 'provided by physicians, hospitals, and pharmacists'.[33] This coincided with the Flexner Report of 1910, which placed restrictions on medical licensure and education. It also helped to establish the hegemony of allopathic medicine at the expense of other forms such as osteopathy and homeopathy.[34] Author and academic Joel Kovel argues that this is the point at which American psychiatry assumed its modern form.[35] This is in line with Foucault's description of how the start of the twentieth century saw clinicians subsuming madness into medicine and thereby justifying the physician's power over the mad.[36] It is noteworthy that Social Phobia was first mentioned by psychiatry around this time.[37]

Psychiatry enjoyed a resurgence in the mid-twentieth century as 'desperate remedies', such as ECT and insulin therapy,[38] were replaced with lithium in 1939; antipsychotics[39] and antidepressants[40] in the 1950s; and benzodiazepines throughout the 1960s and 1970s.[41] All of these were to become dominant modes of treatment for psychiatric diagnoses, with antidepressants still being commonly used for SAD. These psychopharmacological discoveries catalysed the move from institutionalisation to a community-centred model. Not only that, they reinstated the public's trust in psychiatry as having the capability to treat madness[42] and they 'restored psychiatry's wishful identity as a "hard" science'.[43] That is, the biomedical model, which focussed on 'internal mechanism rather than external social factors',[44] offered a means by which psychiatry could stave off encroachment from competing disciplines such as psychology.[45] But psychiatry was not without its critics: the 1960s saw Freudians and antipsychiatrists alike posing a threat to psychiatry's status as a legitimate speciality of medicine.[46] Psychiatrist George Engel, who first established the 'biopsychosocial' model of mental distress,[47] observed that, in response to these threats, it seemed that psychiatrists were imploring of medicine, 'Please take us back and we will never again deviate from the biomedical model.'[48] More recently, in 2010, psychiatrist and president of the American Psychiatric Association (APA), Alan Schatzberg, said that '[w]e need to be more medical to be taken seriously'.[49]

The biomedical model thus serves psychiatry as a 'primary source of its legitimacy as a branch of scientific medicine',[50] and the discipline uses 'complex classifications and statistical procedures to render the appearance of objectivity'.[51] One example of this in action is given by psychiatrist Carl I. Cohen, who describes how the *DSM-III*'s five digit diagnostic codes 'allow for two digits to the right of the decimal point' which gives 'the impression that diagnoses are precise to within one-hundredth of each other'.[52] Paula J. Caplan calls the notion that psychiatric diagnoses are scientific a 'dangerous myth',[53] arguing that they 'do not correspond to clearly identifiable, "real" objects'.[54] Indeed, their diagnostic codes are arbitrary: they cannot be empirically proven nor mathematically derived. Cohen's account of their numbering exemplifies Thomas S. Szasz's tenet that the psy sciences attempt to emulate positivism. These disciplines have typically been viewed as analogous to physics or biology—empirical sciences—when their remit is actually 'moral problems'. This places them outside the domain of science and, by extension, outside the domain of medicine.[55] In striving to emulate empirical sciences, psychiatry has homed in on the biological. The reductionism born of this approach, and what this means for how we conceptualise mental distress, is what I will now explore.

Biological Reductionism

Cohen argues that it is not inherently problematic to explore biological contributors to mental distress since humans are, after all, biological beings.[56] Problems *do* arise, however, when 'psychosocial approaches to mental disorder are eschewed in favor of biological theories and treatments'.[57] This is 'biological reductionism': '[E]xplanations of phenomena occurring at several levels (e.g., social, psychological) that are sought at a single level (biology).'[58] Medical doctor Bruce G. Charlton criticises the very basis of biological models in psychiatry in that they seek to explain the aetiology of mental distress, which is multifaceted, by delving deeper into the brain.[59] Like Cohen, he calls this 'reductionism: the view that the bigger and more complex is explained by the smaller and simpler; and that the smaller and simpler is more fundamental than the bigger and more complex'.[60]

Citing neuroscientist Steven P. R. Rose, Charlton calls these bigger or smaller ways of viewing things 'hierarchical descriptive levels'.[61] At the top of the hierarchy are disciplines such as social psychology and anthropology. We then have psychiatry and behavioural psychology and, as the levels become more fundamental: physiology, chemistry, materials physics, and particle physics. Drawing on the thoughts of philosopher Richard Rorty, Charlton argues that these levels are *not* related in a causal manner, for 'they are simply different ways of describing the same thing'.[62] For the purposes of using biology to explain mental distress, Charlton states that

> [T]o explain psychiatric illness in terms of biochemistry (for example) is not to describe its underlying cause, but to redescribe it.[63] The individual human organism is in question. Either we can describe its abnormal behaviour and how to normalize it in terms of a medical vocabulary (equals psychiatry); or we can describe its cerebral structure, its neurochemical make-up, its pattern of heat distribution, its atomic structure, or whatever we want – but we are not talking about the cause of its behaviour, we are not explaining the behaviour. The organism is unchanged and nothing has been said about causes or explanations.[64]

Engel has argued along similar lines, stating that the biomedical model in psychiatry 'assumes diseases to be fully accounted for by deviations from the norm of measurable biological (somatic) variables. It leaves no room within its framework for the social, psychological, and behavioral dimensions of illness'.[65]

In unduly focussing on the biological, external factors which might contribute to mental distress—*especially* in oppressed groups, such as women—are obfuscated. Yet, this might be the very reason why the biomedical model has enjoyed such popularity. Its occlusion of 'certain aspects of social reality'[66] is reminiscent of what sociologists call the social, or individual, pathology model.[67] This holds that pathology lies within an individual, as opposed to their environment. Academic Angela Thachuk links the social pathology model with the biomedical model by critiquing the way in which '[g]rounding "deviance" in physiological processes'—which Cohen describes as '"drives," instincts, neurochemicals, and genes'[68]—'impedes challenges to [...] sociopolitical norms and context'.[69]

As well as shrouding exogenous contributors to mental distress,[70] biological reductionism provides a 'scientific patina' under which social issues are 'professionalized', 'removed from the realm of public discussion',[71] and placed into the domain of experts.[72] Foucault holds that this is the method by which psychiatry has replaced religious devotion as a means of social control.[73] Cohen elaborates:

> With the decline of religious and political authority, science is one of the few remaining legitimate authorities. Any model that can emulate the scientific methods of the physical sciences lays claim to legitimacy. The use of nosological classifications, esoteric terminology, and statistical procedures give the appearance of objectivity, free of biases of culture or class.[74]

By embracing the biomedical model of mental distress, society has no need to change in the face of social issues and extant structures which breed oppression can continue to thrive. Psychologist Alvin Pam proposes that this interplay has seeped into the very core of biological psychiatry, such that its practitioners engage in 'use of selected data which subtly and unwittingly may represent at times an apologia for existing social structures in the name of "science"'.[75] One such example is the prevalence of homelessness among people experiencing severe mental distress, which biological reductionism would attribute to the mental distress itself, without considering the dearth of affordable homes.[76] Szasz perhaps sums up these apologias in saying that '[w]e now deny moral, personal, political, and social controversies by pretending that they are psychiatric problems'.[77] Caplan has called this '*[t]he psychiatrizing of society*', that is, 'the casting of all negative emotions and difficult behavior as mental illnesses'[78] stemming 'from brain or chemical problems'.[79]

At the time of writing, the biomedical model's popularity does not seem to have waned. Cohen was arguing in the 1990s that the current trend was to view one's personality traits as the result of one's biology: an expression of one's genes.[80] Around the same time, psychiatrist Peter D. Kramer commented on the permeation of biological materialism through our culture, observing that 'newspaper columns, sit-coms, comic strips, talk shows – our public banter is replete with corollaries of the thesis that biology is destiny'.[81] This trend appears to have bled into how we conceptualise mental distress. Writing in 2007, psychologist Michelle N. Lafrance argued that since Depression has been attributed to 'chemical imbalances in the brain',[82] this explanatory model 'has taken hold and currently dominates public opinion of depression',[83] especially in the US.[84] Indeed, the media often 'uncritically'[85] endorses this model, despite—as we shall soon see—evidence as to its validity being lacking.

Thachuk proposes that the root of the proliferation of biological models could lie in their being adopted by mental health advocacy groups in order to reduce stigma.[86] Ironically, the US General Social Survey in 1996 and 2006 found the biomedical model to be 'at best ineffective and at worst potentially stigmatizing'.[87] Clinical psychologist Brett J. Deacon and research scientist Grayson L. Baird propose that this is because it 'foster[s] the perception that the mentally ill lack control over their behavior'.[88] As a result, '[S]uch individuals may be viewed by the public as unpredictable, dangerous, unable to care for themselves, requiring harsher treatment, and fundamentally different from those without mental disorders.'[89]

While the biomedical model does not appear to reduce stigma, it *has* been found to reduce blame.[90] This draws links with sociologist Talcott Parsons's 'sick role'. This concept from medical sociology describes the rights and expectations of the 'sick' individual and becomes relevant in the framing of mental distress as illness. Parsons contends that the sick individual 'cannot be "held responsible" for his condition',[91] nor 'expected by "pulling himself together" to get well [...] he can't "help it"',[92] it is '"not his fault"'.[93] But this absolution comes at a price: Deacon and Baird hold that biological models which conceptualise mental distress as illness 'reinforce concerns about the chronic and untreatable nature of mental disorders'[94] and, in turn, are associated with worse prognoses and 'pessimism about treatment and recovery'.[95]

A subset of the biological model is the 'brain disease' model,[96] which posits that 'mental illnesses' are 'real illnesses of a real organ, the brain'.[97] As the chemical imbalance model has been subject to increasing scrutiny and questioning,[98] even by psychiatrists,[99] so too has attributing mental distress to a diseased brain. For instance, Lisa Appignanesi points out that the post-mortem brains of 'the normal' are remarkably similar to those belonging to people who have experienced mental distress.[100] And even if we accept that mental distress *does* correlate with brain changes, it is difficult, if not impossible, to establish which came first,[101] or which is causative.[102] Appignanesi puts it rather simply: 'I feel sad when my dog dies. That causes a change in my brain. The emotion isn't caused by the brain.'[103]

Conversely, the World Health Organization has claimed that '[w]e know that mental disorders are the outcome of a combination of factors, and that they have a physical basis in the brain'.[104] In response to this, I direct the reader to Deacon's observation that 'scientists have not identified a biological cause of, or even a reliable biomarker for, any mental disorder'.[105] In a similar vein, Pam, writing in 1990, described biological psychiatry's history as

> [A] tale of 'promising leads' [...] that seem to always represent themselves as the long-awaited breakthrough in a steady stream of scientific progress [...] many scholarly assurances that the elusive constitutional mechanism must exist and is just waiting to be discovered [...] rush to print on slender evidence [...] hyperbole as initial reception to new work, and ultimately unproductive results. With each failure, the faith remains undaunted, simply shifting direction in its quest by optimistic lurches from one idea to another. Heuristically, a lot of research has been generated but, following about a century of effort, a harsh assessment would be that no substantive results have been tendered for any 'functional' disorder's pathogenesis.[106]

In 2014, Sami Timimi's assessment of the situation was much the same, for he remarked upon '[t]he failure of decades of basic science research to reveal any specific biological or psychological marker that identifies a psychiatric diagnosis'.[107] If the fruits of biological psychiatry's labour are so lacking, why does it persist in its search? While attempts to reduce stigma and blame might play a part, this is far from the whole story. Enter the pharmaceutical industry.

Big Pharma

While the US might be said to be the global capital of big pharma, the UK is hot on its heels. The UK has the third highest percentage of pharmaceutical research and development expenditure in the world, behind only the US and Japan; one in five of the world's most popular drugs were developed in the UK; proceeds from the pharmaceutical industry form 0.6% of the UK's GDP; and the UK's domestic market is the fifth largest in the world, behind only the US, Japan, Germany, and France. Moreover, a number of leading global pharmaceutical companies—AstraZeneca, GlaxoSmithKline, Eli Lilly—are based in the UK.[108]

Due to UK healthcare being nationalised and US healthcare being privatised, there *are* key differences between the two countries. With that said, some of the issues that plague the US pharmaceutical industry are applicable to the UK, since both house private pharmaceutical companies which are regulated in similar ways. One concern, raised by doctor Peter

Gøtzsche, is that the 1990s and 2000s have seen drug approval policies become more commercially oriented, which has introduced flaws in the production of medical evidence.[109] Although this change has its epicentre in the US, Gøtzsche contends that its ripples are felt globally.

Of the drugs that pharmaceutical companies manufacture, antidepressants (specifically, SSRIs) are of particular relevance since they were the only prescribed drugs that the women in my sample divulged that they had taken for mental distress. Antidepressants gained significant popularity after the US Food and Drug Administration (FDA) approved fluoxetine (Prozac) in 1987, after which it was marketed extensively by Eli Lilly.[110] This surge in popularity has reached further afield than the US and extended to other antidepressants: in 2018, nearly 71 million prescriptions for these drugs were dispensed in the UK, almost double the number prescribed a decade earlier.[111]

In the UK, guidelines to doctors state that individual cognitive behavioural therapy (CBT) should be offered to adults presenting with SAD, with pharmacological interventions being offered if the individual declines CBT or does not obtain adequate relief following it.[112] However, as with NHS treatment in general, and especially for mental health, waiting lists for talking therapies like CBT are long.[113] One in five patients waits longer than a year[114] and, even with the advent of the Improving Access to Psychological Therapies (IAPT) programme,[115] waiting lists can still be several months.[116] Indeed, only 15% of UK residents were able to access IAPT services in 2018.[117] The backlog created by the Covid-19 pandemic has exacerbated the situation,[118] not only in terms of provision of mental healthcare but also the need for it: mental health charity *Mind* reports that 'more people have experienced a mental health crisis during the coronavirus pandemic than ever previously recorded'.[119]

As the wherewithal for providing talking therapies is limited, GPs report being left with no choice but to prescribe medication when the only alternative is a long waiting list.[120] These factors, combined with the nationalisation of healthcare in the UK, create a unique situation. In such a climate of cuts to healthcare[121]—especially mental healthcare[122]—in the name of austerity, and with the added pressure from the pandemic, sociologist Allan Horwitz's observation is cruelly fitting: '[D]rugs [are] clearly both faster and cheaper than years of psychoanalysis.'[123] While some of the women in my sample described how antidepressants had helped them, which I discuss further in Chap. 4, these medications are not without issue. Cohen argues that the actual act of prescribing drugs in psychiatry implies that the problem is solely a biological one, which erases environmental elements[124]—the *opposite* of what this book seeks to do with respect to women and SAD.

But Cohen's tenet is not the only problem with these medications. In England, the number of prescriptions for antidepressants dispensed between 2008 and 2018 doubled.[125] In spite of this, England's *Adult Psychiatric Morbidity Survey 2014* found that overall rates of common mental disorder (CMD)[126] in England have, since 2000, 'steadily increased in women and remained largely stable in men'.[127] Women's mental wellbeing was also disproportionately adversely affected during the pandemic.[128] As levels of mental distress do not seem to be improving and, for women, actually seem to be deteriorating, one might question the efficacy and appropriateness of pharmaceutical treatments such as antidepressants.

This question becomes more pressing when the evidence behind pharmaceuticals' efficacy is reviewed: it appears somewhat scanty, especially given that industry-sponsored trials tend to be of poor quality and are up to 20 times more likely to show higher efficacy than independent and placebo-controlled trials.[129] Physician Ben Goldacre has written an extensive critique of big pharma in the UK, where he contends that poor-quality clinical trials are commonly performed by the same people who manufacture the drugs being trialled. Often, he tells us, the trials are performed in such a way as to skew the results in favour of the drugs' efficacy.[130] Goldacre describes such tactics as 'wily tricks, close calls, and elegant mischief at the margins of acceptability'.[131] Oftentimes, he continues, statistics will be manipulated to make the trials' outcomes seem more promising than they actually are.[132] It is also not unusual for trials to be of inappropriate lengths and sizes; and for new drugs to be compared to drugs not used for the same purpose, in the same way, at the correct dose, or to drugs which are known not to be effective.[133] Results from trials which do not show the 'correct' outcome are simply not published[134] and Goldacre argues that academic papers on a given drug are often written by employees of the companies that manufacture the drug, although this is seldom disclosed.[135]

One of the 'wily tricks' to which Goldacre alludes is examined in more depth by author and academic Irving Kirsch.[136] Kirsch has said that a myriad of data, some of which are hidden by drug companies, demonstrate that antidepressants have no benefit over placebo. When benefits *have* been found, they are below the criterion of 'clinical significance' set by the National Institute for Health and Care Excellence (NICE). What is more, these small benefits over placebo only appear because doctors and/or patients 'break blind':[137] the number of physical side effects which antidepressants can induce, particularly on initiation, allows both doctors and patients to discern who is taking the 'real' drug. And although antidepressants are widely reported to work in clinical practice, by doctors and patients alike, we never see how an individual improves with placebo, by comparison.[138] Furthermore, antidepressants have a number of unpleasant side effects and can cause withdrawal symptoms[139] if stopped.[140] And people who have been treated with them have a greater risk of their mental distress returning than do people who have been treated by other modes.[141]

Discussing *whether* antidepressants work warrants some discussion of *how* they are supposed to work. The purported mechanism connects to the chemical imbalance model, for antidepressants are said to 'correc[t] the neurotransmitter'—usually serotonin[142]—'imbalances that cause mental disorders'.[143] Despite the permeation of the 'low serotonin' model into lay conceptions of mental distress, the consensus in the scientific community seems now to be that this model is not the whole story[144] and is too simplistic.[145] Crucially, Kirsch points out that the benefits conferred by antidepressants occur irrespective of whether they increase or decrease serotonin, or act on another neurotransmitter altogether.[146] On this point, he asks: 'What do you call pills, the effects of which are independent of their chemical composition? I call them "placebos."'[147]

Another issue with antidepressants is their role in diagnostics. As Appignanesi has said, '[T]he girl is said to suffer from depression because she responds to antidepressants.'[148] That therapeutic effect is garnered from a drug is taken to mean that the drug is providing something (usually serotonin) which was hitherto missing, the absence of which was causing the mental distress.[149] In actuality, we do not know whether the drug is acting directly on the mental distress,[150] or in another way altogether.[151] As such, therapeutic effect does not prove either aetiology or that the mental distress has a biological cause.[152] It may come as no surprise, therefore, that the name 'selective serotonin reuptake inhibitor' arose from pharmaceutical marketing as opposed to reflecting a mechanism of action.[153]

On pharmaceutical marketing, psychiatrist Joanna Moncrieff explores an unnamed how-to guide wherein she finds the endorsement of creating 'dissatisfaction in the market', establishing 'a need', and creating 'a desire'.[154] These strategies do not seem compatible with the treatment of legitimate diseases; they seem more akin to medicalising multifaceted problems for economic gain. The words of Paxil's product director, Barry

Brand, are a case in point, for he is quoted as having said that '[e]very marketer's dream [...] is to find an unidentified or unknown market and develop it. That's what we were able to do with social anxiety disorder'.[155]

While SAD has been conceptualised as the medicalisation of shyness,[156] Goldacre has problematised the medicalisation of other normal phenomena. He contends that pharmaceutical companies 'widen the boundaries of diagnosis',[157] and then proffer medicinal 'remedies'. One gendered example is a study on what has been termed 'Female Sexual Dysfunction' (FSD), which claimed that 43% of women were 'affected' by this condition.[158] It later became known that two of the three authors of the paper had worked for the pharmaceutical company Pfizer, which was about to release 'female Viagra'. Their conflict of interest had, of course, not been declared.[159]

The FSD diagnosis has been described by science reporter Denise Grady as the pathologisation of women who do not want sex 'enough', the solution to which can be found in a pill.[160] Sasha Claire McInnes draws our attention to a plethora of other 'conditions' which pathologise women, and for which women are treated, including PMS and Post-traumatic Stress Response to gender-based violence.[161] Pharmaceutical companies therefore are, in the words of McInnes, 'legal drug pushers [...] [who] profit from women's reality'.[162]

These 'legal drug pushers' are regulated by the Medicines and Healthcare Products Regulatory Agency (MHRA) in the UK and the Food and Drug Administration (FDA) in the US. Goldacre puts forth that regulators do not act in the interests of the population but in the interests of the pharmaceutical companies, with this 'regulatory capture' resulting from the crossover of employees.[163] This conflict of interest is analogous to that which exists between biological psychiatry research and the pharmaceutical industry. Pam calls this a '"sleaze" factor' which is introduced into biological psychiatry's research by 'drug money'.[164] For instance, the APA allows pharmaceutical companies, for a price, to sponsor talks at its conferences.[165] As such, the 13*th* World Congress of Psychiatry in 2005 was sponsored by Otsuka Pharmaceutical, Bristol-Myers Squibb, and Eli Lilly.[166] Arrangements such as these have been questioned repeatedly[167] and these challenges are perhaps best summarised by asking, '[H]ow is it that nobody points out the current economic arrangements are inconsistent with scientific objectivity?'[168]

These conflicts of interest mean that the influence of the pharmaceutical industry on psychiatry is pervasive, and some have argued that psychiatric diagnoses and symptoms have 'tailored' themselves to big pharma.[169] Concordant with this, psychiatrist Kramer confesses that the symptoms for which the clinician looks in a patient are contingent on the available drugs.[170] Indeed, as historian Edward Shorter states, 'physicians prefer to diagnose conditions they can treat'[171]—and for which there already exists a pharmaceutical 'cure'—'rather than those they can't'.[172] But what constitutes a psychiatric 'symptom' in need of cure in the first place? We have already seen that psychiatric diagnoses are not scientific, so how are their symptoms determined? Answering these questions requires examining the interplay between 'mental illnesses' and cultural values.

Culture-Bound Syndromes and Cosmetic Psychopharmacology

In *Listening to Prozac*, psychiatrist Kramer chronicles his observations after prescribing the antidepressant Prozac to several individuals over a number of years. In so doing, he characterises a number of these individuals as 'good responders'.[173] And although Kirsch's tenets on antidepressants and the placebo effect are convincing, psychiatrist James Warner makes a point pertinent to Kramer's findings in stating that '[l]ooking at mean responses irons out those that don't respond at all and those that respond quite well'.[174]

One of Kramer's key insights in *Listening to Prozac* is that the category 'mental illness' is strongly contingent on the norms and demands of the prevailing culture. He explains:

> Seeing how poorly patients fared when they were cautious and inhibited, and how the same people flourished once medication had made them assertive and flexible, I developed a strong impression of how our culture favors one interpersonal style over another.[175]

Some people, Kramer argues, only 'need' psychiatric or pharmacologic treatment because their environments do not favour their traits or temperament.[176] Of particular relevance is that a lot of Kramer's case studies' traits are consistent with social anxiety. For instance, he speaks of one person's experience of rejections: Kramer characterises these as arising not due to the patient's inability, but due to 'various institutions' prejudice in favor of extraversion and "assertiveness"'.[177] On this point, Christopher Lane questions 'whether "social phobia" and "avoidant personality disorder" may at times represent a type of noncompliance with our culture's demand for extroversion'.[178] Another of Kramer's case studies 'became [...] more assertive socially' after taking Prozac,[179] while another still said that Prozac 'makes me confident'.[180] A further individual 'became socially capable, no longer a wallflower but a social butterfly'.[181]

Kramer thus observes that Prozac makes people 'socially attractive':[182] it is able 'to give social confidence to the habitually timid, to make the sensitive brash, to lend the introvert the social skills of a salesman'.[183] In discussing one particular individual, Sally, Kramer posits that her mental distress arose from the social inhibition in her temperament as opposed to illness. This then begs the question of what Prozac is actually medicating when it is administered to somebody like Sally, and Kramer queries whether it is not her very personality which is being changed.[184] If this is the case, does medicating for SAD 'cure' the normal personality trait of shyness? Kramer dubs such medicating 'cosmetic psychopharmacology',[185] that is, the 'reshaping of personality traits by medication'.[186] If medications like Prozac are indeed altering aspects of personality 'that might have succeeded in a different, and not especially distant, culture',[187] we ought then to question its purpose: is it to cure, to treat, or to make people conform to what the dominant culture values?

The idea that Prozac medicates people to conformity draws links with the thoughts of Peter Conrad on biomedical enhancement.[188] Indeed, Kramer points out that a significant number of the people he has found to be rendered 'better than well'[189] by Prozac have had what he calls 'mild degrees of impairment: minor depression, minor compulsiveness, sensitivity to loss, personality styles fallen from favour'.[190] These people only 'need' treatment because of 'how exigent our culture is in its behavioral demands'.[191]

Following Kramer, we can see that psychiatric diagnoses are strongly rooted in cultural norms. A prime example is addressed by psychiatrist Richard S. Schwartz in discussing antidepressant use for 'prolonged' bereavement.[192] In the US, 'prolonged' is a year after the bereavement; in rural Greece, it is usual for relatives of the deceased to grieve for five years. Schwartz thus suggests that medicating with 'mood brighteners' can potentially to be used to justify and reinforce oppressive cultural norms and expectations.

Given that what is classed as 'mental illness', and what warrants pharmacologic treatment, is entangled with culture, the concept of the 'culture-bound syndrome' (CBS) is salient. Academic Ivan Crozier defines CBSs as follows: '[A] group of symptoms (mental, physical, social) that is recognized within a specific culture, with accepted treatments within these cultures. Such illnesses are not universal; they are not caused by other neurological or psychiatric conditions.'[193] The notion of a CBS, though not called by this name, had been discussed for many years prior to its inclusion in the *DSM* in 1994. It has its origins in the colonial psychiatry of the nineteenth and early twentieth centuries, owing to figures such as psychiatrist Emil Kraepelin's observations of phenomena such as *koro* (briefly, the belief and resulting panic that the penis is shrinking into the abdomen) in East Asia.

Kraepelin understood CBSs not to be 'separate diseases'.[194] Rather, he believed that all people suffered from the same diseases, but that 'culture' altered a disease's presentation. Kraepelin's legacy is still visible in contemporary psychiatry in the way that CBSs are often conceptualised.[195] Presumably in response to criticisms of the way that CBSs had been included in the *DSM*, the APA released an addendum to the *DSM-5* in 2013. This document states that the 'DSM-5 [*sic*] updates criteria to reflect cross-cultural variations in presentations',[196] with the following given as an example: '[U]ncontrollable crying and headaches are symptoms of panic attacks in some cultures, while difficulty breathing may be the primary symptom in other cultures.'[197] Although the addendum claims that the *DSM* 'incorporates a greater cultural sensitivity',[198] it is clear that it endorses Kraepelin's viewpoint that CBSs are, at root, the same 'disorders', with 'culture' altering their presentations.

Rather than situating *all* mental distress in its cultural context, the *DSM* seems to define CBSs in terms of their Western 'equivalents'. An example of this can be found in how it deals with the Japanese phenomenon *taijin kyofusho*, which concerns a person's 'fear that they will displease or embarrass others'.[199] The *DSM-5* incorporates 'fear of "offending others"' into its criteria for SAD in order 'to reflect the Japanese concept in which avoiding harm to others is emphasized'.[200] The *DSM-5* thus effectively subsumes *taijin kyofusho* into SAD, implicitly saying that they are the same disease entity, manifested differently due to 'culture'. As anthropologist Charles C. Hughes has argued of the *DSM-IV*, culture should not merely be '"taken into account" off-handedly as a side issue (as repeatedly suggested in DSM-IV [*sic*])'.[201] Conversely, Hughes puts forth that culture is 'embedded in the culturally structured scenario between the patient and clinician, no matter where it occurs'.[202] On this point, Cohen invites the reader to imagine the decisions and assessments a clinician needs to make before diagnosing a patient as being paranoid. That is, the clinician needs to assess the patient's behaviour contextually—in light of cultural norms and practices—in order to ascertain whether it is reasonable.[203]

Crozier makes a further critique of the *DSM*'s treatment of CBSs, namely that their placement—in appendices[204]—and description therein reveals an ethnocentrism.[205] He points out 'the privileged position' of Western psychiatry, which thinks of itself as being 'beyond culture'.[206] This is evident in its conceptualisation of *koro* cases in the West: in positing that *koro* is possible 'out of cultural context',[207] it implies 'that culture is elsewhere (i.e., nonwestern)'.[208] Of course, the West *does* have cultural context, and Hughes argues that culture is 'just as much a factor in shaping particular patterns of symptomatology in Western societies as it is everywhere else'.[209] He therefore suggests that *all* diagnostic categories should address cultural context, and proposes introducing the category 'Western CBSs'. This would incorporate diagnoses such as 'post-traumatic stress disorder, dissociative identity disorder' and, most relevant for this book, 'social phobia'.[210] Hughes also views Western CBSs through a gendered lens in making the case that diagnoses such as Pre-menstrual Syndrome, Body Dysmorphic Disorder, Anorexia Nervosa, and Bulimia Nervosa be considered in light of 'cultural beliefs about ideal body shape, sexuality and women's societal roles in Western societies'.[211]

Since cultural context is inextricable from psychiatric diagnosis, the temporal and the geographical are of utmost importance. As Crozier concludes from considering *koro*, some diagnoses exist 'only at a certain time and place'.[212] This relates to Kramer's observation that mental distress can result from possessing certain temperaments which, though they may have been rewarded in a bygone era, are no longer valued by an individual's containing culture. To explore this as it pertains to women, we must briefly chart the evolution of contemporary ideals of femininity vis-à-vis personality style.

Sociologist Kathy Deliovsky tells us that 'idealized representations of white femininity occurred in distinct historical phases within the context of European colonialism/slavery and imperialism'.[213] She writes of 'idealized representations [which] portray[ed] white women as bathed [in] and permeated by white light'.[214] That is,

> [G]lowing representation was constructed alongside their positioning as the moral custodians and bearers of the white race. White women were accorded a position of moral superiority above all non-Anglo-Saxon women and at the same time were contained within rigid identities/categories of virtuous lady and mother [...] white women's image signifies the apogee of beauty, motherhood and morality.[215]

The religious and moral threads which run through Deliovsky's description evoke 'The Angel in the House',[216] a Victorian poem describing the ideal woman of that time: wife, mother, and cornerstone of family life. In the words of Virginia Woolf, the Angel was

> [I]mmensely sympathetic, immensely charming, utterly unselfish. She excelled in the difficult arts of family life. She sacrificed herself daily [...] if there was a draught she sat in it [...] she was so constituted that she never had a mind but preferred to sympathize always with the minds and wishes of others [...] Her purity was supposed to be her chief beauty.[217]

Femininities are, of course, many; contingent on time and place; and infused with other axes of oppression such as race and class.[218] And while ideals have shifted since the Angel, the legacy of ideal Victorian femininity can be seen in late twentieth and early twenty-first-century UK and US contexts insofar as 'behaviour and decorum in service of white masculinity'[219] are still highly valued.

Exactly what constitutes this behaviour and decorum can be learned by visiting the work of psychologist Sandra Bem who, in 1974, formed the Bem Sex Role Inventory. This comprises traits which were 'judged to be more desirable [in American society] for a woman than for a man'.[220] Echoing the Victorian 'Angel', the Inventory deemed a person to be 'feminine' if they could be described as: affectionate, cheerful, childlike, compassionate, not using harsh language, eager to soothe hurt feelings, flatterable, gentle, gullible, loving children, loyal, sensitive to the needs of others, shy, soft spoken, sympathetic, tender, understanding, warm, and yielding.[221]

Since Bem's Inventory, the ideal has evolved. Writing in 1993, Kramer alludes to the personality style in favour for women at that time in citing '[v]ivacious women's attractiveness to men' and 'men's discomfort with anhedonia in women'.[222] But in contrast with the Victorian ideal, Kramer tells us that the 1990s saw traditionally 'masculine' traits valued in women:

'[R]esilience, energy, assertiveness, [and] an enjoyment of give-and-take'.[223] This reflected wider social change in the decades preceding Kramer's opus, particularly the late 1970s and early 1980s, such as more individualistic politics and an increasing number of women working outside of the home. As feminist cultural theorist Rosalind Gill notes, it was in this period that 'notions of male and female equality and the basic similarity of men and women took hold in popular culture'.[224]

As I am writing in 2023, the past 30 years have seen the ideal develop further. This might be attributed to the feminist movement's call for parity with men; indeed, a woman exhibiting masculine traits is now more acceptable than ever.[225] As such, my conception of the current ideal personality style for women is derived from Victorian femininity, but bears resemblance to the femininity described by Kramer: I will call this 'masculine femininity'. Broadly, this can be thought of as traditional femininity—as found in the 'Angel' and described by Bem's Inventory—with the addition of typically masculine traits which are valued in contemporary UK and US culture. These include being ambitious, assertive, independent, competitive, individualistic, self-reliant, self-sufficient, and having leadership abilities.[226]

In addition to considering Gill's remarks on wider social change, we can understand why trends in femininity have shifted thus by looking to the work of trans theory writer Julia Serano. Serano observes that, in our patriarchal society, masculinity is valued more than femininity. Hence, women's wanting to espouse masculine characteristics is seen as understandable. On the contrary, men's wanting to exhibit feminine traits counters the idea that men are superior, and so tends not to be tolerated—think about how girls playing with toy cars are accepted more readily than boys playing with Barbie dolls.[227] Building on Serano's observations, I argue that women's exhibiting masculine traits is not merely tolerated, but is now *expected*. At the same time, the Victorian legacy of femininity still bears weight. As such, women face the unreasonable expectation that they display opposite and incompatible traits: for example, assertiveness (masculine) and shyness (feminine).

Relating this back to the thoughts of Kramer, one of his arguments is that women exhibiting traits of the Victorian ideal are not rewarded in today's society, leading to a 'mismatch between women's coping style and the requisites for finding reward in this culture'.[228] Given that Victorian styles of femininity undeniably inform today's ideal, this seems a little simplistic: *some* feminine traits are still valued in women, even if masculine traits are now valued too. With that said, his argument still has utility. In seeing individuals' personality traits altered by Prozac, Kramer proposes that the drug can change 'overly-feminine'[229] traits,[230] such as passivity—or indeed, social anxiety—to those which the culture values in women: assertiveness and spiritedness. In so doing, Kramer questions whether we are not endorsing 'a certain sort of social conformity':[231] in bringing women into line with '"masculine" capitalist values',[232] does Prozac serve the economic needs of society?

Kramer thus wonders whether Prozac is akin to drugs such as Miltown, Librium, and Valium: the 'mother's little helpers' of the 1960s and 1970s. These drugs were used to keep women in their place in society and make them content with the drudgery of housework. As psychiatrist Jonathan M. Metzl explains, '[T]he pills became known as the treatments of choice for the pressures of motherhood, single-hood and other historically specific forms of essentialised womanhood.'[233] By contrast, Kramer cites the experience of one individual, Julia, for whom Prozac 'got [her] out of the house and into the workplace, where she was able to grow in competence and confidence'.[234] Kramer hence describes antidepressants as 'feminist drugs, liberating and empowering'.[235] But is Prozac *really* the antithesis of the mother's little helpers of yesteryear? Or, as Serano might argue, is it more acceptable since it nurtures *masculine* traits in women? In attempting to answer this, it is worth considering that psychopharmaceuticals have been described as a 'woman's best friend' in terms of 'dealing with the pressures of working in a man's world'.[236] Perhaps, as the demands to which women are subject have changed, so too have the drugs which enable them to cope.

This calls to mind a study cited by Schwartz which finds that people who are depressed are better at predicting probabilities than people who are not. Since the non-depressed are 'too optimistic',[237] we might say that the depressed have a more realistic perspective of the world. Medicating these people then reduces their ability to predict probabilities and, by extension, disconnects them from the bleakness of reality. This evokes McInnes's likening of pharmacological interventions such as antidepressants to the 'soma' of Aldous Huxley's *Brave New World*:

> And if ever, by some unlucky chance, anything unpleasant should somehow happen, why, there's always soma to give you a holiday from the facts. And there's always soma to calm your anger, to reconcile you to your enemies, to make you patient and long suffering.[238]

Continuing with this dystopian thread, Kramer imagines a society where a plethora of emotions and personality traits are medicated:

> 'Why such a long face? Can't you take a MoodStim before work?' A family doctor warns the widow, 'If you won't try AntiGrief, we'll have to consider hospitalization.' And a parent urges the paediatrician to put a socially anxious child on AntiWallflower Compound.[239]

While these examples are extreme (and, of course, fictional), I invite the reader to consider the salience of their undergirding principles for medicating different forms of mental distress—especially social anxiety in women.

In drawing this section to a close, I want to bring together the two schools of thought which inform the book's theoretical approach: anti-psychiatry and feminism. McInnes points to these movements having had a bifurcated history: she argues that just as psychiatry (and, I would add, anti-psychiatry) has not generally acknowledged feminism, 'The feminist movement has not yet embraced "madwomen".'[240] While McInnes raises a valid point, there *are* literatures which have successfully drawn upon these two approaches, many of which deal with overtly gendered diagnoses—Pre-menstrual Dysphoric Disorder (PMDD), Pre-menstrual Syndrome (PMS), Female Sexual Dysfunction (FSD), and Postpartum Depression (PPD). Therefore, in the second half of this chapter, I explore common threads which emerge from this existing research and outline how this book's analysis of women's SAD will borrow from and build upon it.

Cultural Values, (Ab)normality, and Medicalising Difference

As my eschewing of a solely biomedical model of mental distress might suggest, this book takes a social constructionist approach. For the purposes of the book's remit, this perspective holds that psychiatric diagnosis is contingent on, and shaped by, culture.[241] Gendered psychiatric diagnoses are especially ripe for being viewed through this lens, as sociologist Kathy Kendall demonstrates in her writing on Pre-menstrual Syndrome (PMS)—an exaggerated version of which features in the *DSM-5* as Pre-menstrual Dysphoric Disorder (PMDD).[242] Kendall makes the case that probing the scientific institution which uses a 'disease model' to conceptualise women's monthly cycles reveals 'a social, political and gendered institution which reflects cultural concepts, values, ideologies and practices'.[243] According to academics Kirsten K. Johnson and Mary-Anne Kandrack, it follows that science 'contains and maintains perspectives of the social order'.[244]

Other authors have also interrogated the social construction of PMS.[245] Women's health activist and writer Esther Rome has explored how even PMS's specific *symptoms* 'take on a value influenced by society'. For instance, bloating 'would not carry a social stigma if we [...] believed fatness was beautiful'.[246] I invite the reader to apply Rome's tenet to social anxiety. If its physical manifestations, such as blushing and hand tremor,[247] were viewed as attractive, how would socially anxious women view their experiences? Would they seek psychiatric help for them? This calls to mind Ussher's contention that we 'do not experience symptoms in a sociocultural vacuum':[248] they cannot be understood in a standalone manner,[249] for they are dependent on cultural and historical context.[250] This evokes the CBS and, in line with Hughes's ideas, several feminist authors have conceptualised PMDD as such.[251]

Since psychiatric 'symptoms' depend on cultural and historical context, psychologists Joan C. Chrisler and Paula J. Caplan[252] question whether the line between 'normal' and 'abnormal' can ever definitively be drawn. Similarly, sociologist Natasha Mauthner argues that the medical establishment's conceptualisation of postnatal depression as 'illness'[253] produces 'a false dichotomy': there is a 'normal' state, where motherhood is a wholly positive experience, and a 'pathological' state of Postnatal Depression.[254] Instead of this dichotomy, Women's Studies scholar Chloë Taylor argues that 'the pathological is on a hazy continuum with the banal'.[255] This tenet has been applied to other gendered psychiatric diagnoses, with philosopher Cressida Heyes contending that 'there is no "bright line" between Body Dysmorphic Disorder and "normal" feminine preoccupations with physical appearance'.[256] Feminist psychotherapist and author Susie Orbach makes a comparable point in writing that 'there is a painful continuity between most women's daily experience and that of the anorectic woman. Nearly all women feel the necessity to restrain their appetites and diminish their size'.[257]

Considering Taylor's hazy continuum in the case of SAD begs the following question: at what point, if ever, is shyness or social anxiety pathological? Even the *DSM* task forces collating SAD's diagnostic criteria in the 1980s grappled with this conundrum, since '[a] few experts insisted they wanted to treat only "extreme shyness,"[258] but others admitted they were unable to distinguish between that trait and Social Anxiety Disorder'.[259] So, they were put on the same spectrum, with the co-authors of *Social Anxiety Disorder: A Guide* explaining with surprising nonchalance, 'Where shyness ends and social anxiety disorder begins isn't clear. Some social anxiety is expected in everyone.'[260]

Taylor writes further on the notion of a continuum, suggesting that traditionally feminine traits are deemed to be abnormal when they are extreme—think about Kramer's descriptor of passivity as an 'overly-feminine'[261] trait which can be medicated. In the words of Taylor, '[T]he pathological is not so much opposed to the norm as the norm exaggerated.'[262] Since masculine traits are viewed as the default, feminine traits are already deemed abnormal. Their exaggerated form is then seen as doubly aberrant. This brings us to norms of femininity, and the part that they play in psychiatric diagnoses.

Ussher explores how the PMDD diagnosis hinges on gendered traits, for it can be diagnosed in women with the 'feminised' pre-menstrual symptoms of 'anxiety, tearfulness, and depression'.[263] Similarly, what started life as 'hysterical personality disorder', and was in 1980 renamed 'histrionic personality disorder',[264] has been described by author Mary Ann Jimenez as 'essentially a caricature of exaggerated femininity'.[265] Its symptoms consist of 'excitability, emotional instability, over-reactivity and self-dramatisation'.[266] A person likely to be diagnosed with this might be 'someone who is "typically attractive and seductive ... overly concerned with physical attractiveness" as well as interested in "control(ling) the opposite sex or enter(ing) into a dependent relationship (and continuously demanding) reassurance, approval or praise"'.[267] Ussher asks of this description: 'Isn't this how we are taught to "do girl" through teenage magazines, romantic fiction, and "chick flicks? [*sic*]'.[268] Relating this to SAD, sociologist Erving Goffman claims that women are 'socialized [...] to project "shyness"' and '"reserve"'.[269] These diagnoses then exemplify a cruel contradiction: women are socialised into behaving according to norms of femininity and—since these norms are inherent in certain diagnoses—in doing so are pathologised.

Taylor provides commentary on women's pathologisation in broader terms by questioning the disease status of several diagnoses which come under the 'Female Sexual Dysfunction' (FSD) umbrella: Female Orgasmic Disorder,[270] Female Sexual Interest/Arousal Disorder,[271] and Genito-Pelvic Pain/Penetration Disorder.[272] Taylor points out that the National

Health and Social Life Survey of 1999[273] claimed that 32% of women had Hypoactive Sexual Desire Disorder[274] and that this number rose to more than 50% in women over 40.[275] She then makes the case that these women's 'symptoms' are, in a statistical sense, normal.[276] Taylor thus not only doubts whether FSD is a psychiatric disorder,[277] but, since it is *statistically* normal, she proposes that it has been conceptualised as being 'abnormal in some *other* way — such as ideologically'.[278] '[T]he ideological norm in question', she tells us, 'is a medical construction of female sexuality tailored to appeal to modern, Western, heterosexual men'.[279]

Bringing Taylor's argument to bear on SAD, the *DSM-5*'s definition of this diagnosis comprises '[m]arked fear or anxiety about one or more social situations in which the individual is exposed to possible scrutiny by others'.[280] An example of this situation writ large is public speaking, and this phobia has been construed within the psy science literature as a subtype of SAD.[281] Indeed, the *DSM-5*'s diagnostic criteria state that physicians should '*[s]pecify* if: Performance only: If the fear is restricted to speaking or performing in public'.[282] As Taylor points to the prevalence of FSD in questioning its validity as an illness, let us do the same for nervousness about public speaking. A US community sample found its rate to be 20.6%;[283] another found it to occur in one in three people;[284] and a further US community survey put the figure at 55%.[285] If we are not to restrict ourselves to public speaking, but consider social anxiety more broadly, author of *Shyness: What It Is, what To Do about It* Philip G. Zimbardo suggests that around 90% of people have experienced social anxiety symptoms.[286] It is also worth pointing out that none of the above cited studies differentiate between genders. Given that SAD appears to be more common in women,[287] the prevalence of public speaking phobia—or indeed social anxiety more broadly—is likely higher in women than these studies indicate: statistically, it may be normal. Recall Kramer's discussion of the way in which our culture prefers certain traits in women: 'Vivacious women's attractiveness to men'[288] and 'resilience, energy, assertiveness, [and] an enjoyment of give-and-take'.[289] Since socially anxious women are not likely to exhibit these traits, I wonder if their social anxiety, like FSD, is not abnormal *statistically*, but has been conceptualised as being abnormal *ideologically*.

Caplan makes an argument connected to statistical normality in critiquing Eli Lilly's medication Sarafem. Sarafem is Prozac, repackaged in pink and purple casing, and marketed to women for PMS/PMDD. Caplan comments on the explanatory materials for Sarafem, arguing that Eli Lilly have

> [A]dded a list of mood problems from the PMDD list that virtually every human being experiences. Even the National Institute of Mental Health website muddies the distinction between PMS and PMDD. This is called 'category creep,' a way of deeming increasing numbers of people mentally ill.[290]

Following Zimbardo, given that social anxiety is also something that virtually every human being experiences, it is worth asking whether SAD is also subject to category creep. But category creep deems people to be mentally unwell not only by conceptualising arguably normal experiences as illness, but by conceptualising diverse behaviours as problems which, in turn, are medicalised.

Rome writes on the latter in the case of PMS. She criticises what she sees as the tendency of some feminists to claim that the majority of women are 'normal', with but a few experiencing disruption pre-menstrually. This, she claims, 'serves to separate those who "pass" in our male regulated society from those who can't or won't pass, rather than to examine the broader issues of societal rules not classifying a wider range of human experience as acceptable'.[291] Bioethicist and philosopher of medicine Tamara Kayali Browne relates this to the feminine ideal, contending that its existence 'discourage[s] acceptance of variations in female behaviour'.[292] Browne proposes that one of the ways by which the acceptance of diverse behaviours is discouraged is through labelling them as 'disorders' which, in turn, legitimises treatments. On the other hand, if a *difference* were to be regarded as simply that—consider, for our purposes, shyness—then 'treatment' would be seen as unethical, even harmful.[293]

Taking this argument a step further, we have the idea that difference should not merely be tolerated, but that it might actually be positive. Browne cites cases of Depression which have acted as a 'catalyst for change'[294] insofar as they signified that something had 'gone awry' in people's lives.[295] Browne adds that '[a] similar argument has been made for anxiety in social situations [...]—that such reactions are normal and can even be useful'.[296]

Erica Leibrandt, a psychotherapist and author who identifies as a 'Socially Anxious Person', fleshes out Browne's remark in describing some of the benefits of social anxiety. These include saving energy for 'things that are really important to us', namely social gatherings; having a tendency to be compassionate, empathetic, and tolerant of others' quirks, owing to our own; being incredibly loyal once we find friends who we trust; having learned to enjoy solitude; and, due to finding a lot of situations stressful, not taking things for granted.[297] Leibrandt's perspective stands in stark contrast to the rather hopeless picture presented by the Royal College of Psychiatrists's resource on 'Shyness and Social Phobia', which tells us that

> Many sufferers cope by arranging their lives around their symptoms.
> This means that they (and their families) have to miss out on things they might otherwise enjoy.
> They can't visit their children's school, can't do the shopping or go to the dentist. They may even actively avoid promotion at work, even though they are quite capable of doing a more demanding and more financially rewarding job.
> About half of those with a severe phobia, particularly men, will have difficulty in making long-term relationships.[298]

Philosopher Jacquelyn Zita draws attention to an analogous picture when considering women's monthly cycles. Although many women across several studies attest that their midcycle is a time of heightened mood, productivity, and creativity,[299] this is seldom given attention: it does not comport with the dominant narrative which instead focuses on the 'time of the month' as being 'a time of illness and dysphoria'.[300] But what *are* these dominant narratives? From where do they arise? How do they form? And what do they do to our experiences? To address these questions, we must look to the social construction of 'mental illness'.

Dominant Narratives and the Social Construction of 'Mental Illness'

Ussher's research on women and PMDD exemplifies how dominant narratives shape our experiences of mental distress. That is, she found that when her participants were asked to describe their PMS, they

> [R]e-produced the key symptoms found in academic and popular texts on PMDD [...] describing, and simultaneously interpreting, their premenstrual bodily and psychological experiences within the narrow symptom checklist model of PMDD presented by the psychiatry/psychology professions.[301]

Ussher's work points to individuals' narratives being shaped by both diagnostic criteria and the psychiatric and popular discourses which these diagnostic criteria spur. Chrisler and Caplan elaborate on the latter, drawing our attention to the prominence of the figure of the pre-menstrual woman in popular culture, beginning around 1980. Women's narratives of their own experiences then inevitably become influenced by this stereotype.[302] And while the figure of the *socially anxious* woman is not so ubiquitous, the hegemony of biological psychiatry means that the figure of the socially anxious woman with an 'illness like any other' is perhaps beginning to gain a foothold.

The points made by Ussher are merged with those of Chrisler and Caplan by Science and Technology Studies scholar Judy Segal in discussing psychiatry's identification and treatment of FSD. She notes that professional,[303] corporate,[304] and popular[305] forces are confluent in 'persuad[ing] women that low desire is abnormal and may be a sign of biological disease'.[306] She continues:

> We all experience distress in the terms available for us to experience it in [...] We are surrounded by professional and public discourses — rhetorics — about health and illness. These rhetorics are imbued with values [...] We absorb these values and draw on them in interpreting our own experience of health and illness.[307]

Segal thus proposes exploring the means by which our distress is presented to us as being 'best thought of as contained in our individual bodies, expressing a disease, in need of a drug'.[308] Segal's remarks allude to repudiating the biological model of mental distress and interrogating the social construction of 'mental illness'. It is crucial at this juncture to state that this does *not* mean denying women's mental distress or dispossessing them of their experiences. To this end, I agree with academic Lisa Cosgrove's theorising of PMS, for she posits that 'the materiality of premenstrual change [is] discursively constructed and experienced as PMS or PMDD in particular socio-cultural contexts, and premenstrual distress [develops] in the context of women's lives'.[309]

With that said, it is equally crucial to examine *why* psychiatry presents certain experiences as pathological. In the case of PMS, Ussher posits that this 'disease' emerged in the wake of greater gender equality in the West. That is, '[T]he belief that women are erratic and unreliable premenstrually serv[ed] to restrict women's access to equal opportunities'[310]—notably, it restricted their access to certain professions, for example, working as presidents,[311] doctors, and pilots.[312] PMS's being conceptualised as a mental disorder thus maintained, and arguably continues to maintain, the status quo by perpetuating women's inequality.[313] Analogously, we might put forth that social anxiety in women is classified as a mental disorder because the socially anxious woman contravenes the ideals of femininity which serve our neoliberal and postfeminist society.

In examining the social construction of PMS, another facet which comes to the fore is emotion. Several feminist writers have posited that women 'allow'[314] themselves to display emotion—frustration, listlessness, anger—pre-menstrually[315] because doing so is 'culturally sanctioned'.[316] That is, these emotions can be expressed on the proviso that they are attributed to 'a medical condition' (PMS),[317] for this allows the 'social conditions'[318] which might be causing these emotions to remain buried.[319] In addition, it serves a purpose for the individual woman. As Caplan explains: 'It seems less daunting to say, "It must be hormonal!" than to begin the frightening process of looking at underlying causes and realising, for instance, "I need to leave this job — or relationship."'[320] Following this, Ussher contends that positioning 'premenstrual negative affect as "not me"'[321] allows a woman to 'avoid an assault on the self'.[322] This 'dualistic discourse'—'Jekyll & Hyde, "me/not me," "PMS-self/real-self"'—has proliferated to such an extent that Chrisler has found it to feature in many PMS self-help books.[323] And in much the same way that Ussher observed how women's descriptions of their PMS echoed psychiatric symptom checklists, a number of studies have found dualistic discourse in the narratives of (heterosexual) women themselves.[324]

As attributing negative affect to PMS can protect a woman's view of her self and her circumstances, Chrisler and Caplan describe how attributing 'unfeminine' traits or behaviours to PMS can permit women 'to hold onto a self-definition of "good/proper" woman'.[325] In so doing, women can 'aspire to the ideal without having to admit that it is impossible to achieve'.[326] While Chrisler and Caplan frame this as a coping mechanism, Ussher and Perz argue that the dissonance between reality and 'idealised cultural constructions' actually *contributes* to women's Depression.[327] Mauthner makes a concordant point in proposing that PPD 'arises out of the discrepancy' that mothers experience 'between the mother they want to be and the mother they feel they are'[328]—a point we might extrapolate to other forms of mental distress, like SAD, if 'mother' is replaced by 'woman'.

Whether divorcing difficult emotions from ourselves reduces or exacerbates mental distress, Ussher contends that, in doing so, '[W]e foster a sense of alienation or distance from ourselves.'[329] In turn, we measure ourselves against 'an idealised construction of femininity'.[330] This comparison is carried out using self-surveillance, a phenomenon which I have linked to women's experiences of SAD elsewhere[331] and one which warrants further exploration. To do so, we must map its origins.

Self-Surveillance and Self-Silencing

Whereas I have drawn upon Foucault's *History of Madness*[332] thus far, it is to another of his works, *Discipline and Punish*,[333] that I now turn. Therein, Foucault explores self-surveillance using philosopher Jeremy Bentham's Panopticon. This 'perfect prison' is a cylindrical building comprised of abutting cells about a central watchtower. There is an inmate in each cell, however they cannot see each other; thus an inmate is unable to be a 'subject of communication'.[334] This prevents mutiny because organising such requires communication. As a result, the inmates' compliance is ensured. Because only the central observation point, and not what or who is inside, is visible from the cells, the inmates do not know whether they are being observed at any given time. The configuration is thus 'a machine for dissociating the see/being seen dyad'[335] and hence gives rise to inmates' *behaving as though they are being observed, irrespective of whether they are or not*. The result is a very effective and efficient disciplinary model, since the tower can be unstaffed. Consequently, the inmates essentially watch themselves: they engage in self-surveillance and, by extension, self-regulation. The inmates have, Foucault tells us, internalised the 'inspecting' gaze of the surveyor: '[A] gaze which each individual under its weight will end by interiorising to the point that he is his own overseer; each individual thus exercising the surveillance over, and against, himself. A superb formula, power exercised continuously.'[336]

As to this concept's relevance for gendered psychiatric diagnoses, Ussher and Perz, in their research on PMS, find some of their participants to be 'engaging in self-surveillance'.[337] That is, these women measure their own needs against cultural constructions of the ideal woman who is 'responsible, self-renunciating, and always able to offer unlimited care and attention to others'.[338] This links to the way that women are positioned as being solely responsible for their relationships[339] and how they must, as Caplan notes, 'maintain closeness with others, regardless of the cost to themselves'.[340] The words of feminist philosopher Jean Grimshaw are salient here, for she states that 'not upsetting people must always be given priority' for women[341]—something which especially rings true for *socially anxious* women.

Ussher and Perz allude to Grimshaw's remark in their study on women and PMS. When the women in their sample expressed negative emotions within their relationships, they became subject to their 'inner critics'. The inner critic is a self that is 'surveillant, judging [...] vigilant',[342] resonating both with the self-surveillance and the 'me, not me' duality on which I touched earlier. But a third, related, concept arises from these literatures on women's mental distress: self-silencing.

Ussher and Perz propose that women experiencing PMS are in fact engaging in self-silencing: it is not that they become angry or irritable once per month; rather, they *suppress* these emotions for the rest of the month.[343] PMS is then conceptualised as 'ruptures' in this self-silencing.[344] Self-silencing originates in the work of psychologist Dana Crowley Jack who linked this phenomenon to women's Depression[345] and produced *The Silencing the Self Scale*.[346] In Jack's schema, 'silencing the self' is described as 'the inhibition of thoughts and feelings to avoid relationship conflict and loss'.[347] For the socially anxious woman, silencing the self might also preserve others' favourable impressions.

Most relevant for this work is what Jack, along with fellow psychologist Diana Dill, calls the 'divided self': '[B]ehaving in a compliant manner to live up to female role imperatives whilst feeling angry inside.'[348] These female role imperatives are reminiscent of the self-surveillance-fostering cultural constructions of ideal womanhood about which Ussher and Perz write. Crucially, Jack and Dill's 'divided self' is also reminiscent of Laing's conception of the self in his opus of the same name.[349] Indeed, I have linked Laing's 'divided self' to women's social anxiety elsewhere,[350] and I will explore his work in more depth in Chap. 6. But while Laing's *The Divided Self* is arguably his best known work, he is famously quoted as having described insanity as 'a perfectly rational adjustment to an insane world'.[351] It is this tenet that I now discuss.

'Mental Illnesses' as Rational Responses and the Medicalisation of Distress

Several feminist scholars' writings echo Laing's tenet in considering the role that women's inequality plays in their mental distress. Psychologist Janet Stoppard has described women's Depression as being 'a result of the gendered power imbalance in a patriarchal society',[352] while Ussher reframes the irritability of women with children, supposedly arising from PMS, as 'a legitimate response to lack of partner support in the home'.[353] Chrisler and Johnston-Robledo also speak to this notion in emphasising the role that 'the stress of women's busy, overburdened lives and, in some cases, traumatic events' play in PMS.[354]

On Chrisler and Johnston-Robledo's latter point, Browne tells us that since '[w]omen experience disproportionate levels of stress and trauma in comparison to men [...] it is not surprising that they suffer from disproportionate levels of psychological distress'.[355] Ussher has written on a particularly gendered example, sexual violence, from which many women diagnosed with Borderline Personality Disorder have suffered as children.[356] Far from being pathology, Ussher puts forth that these women's anger is a justifiable response to what has happened to them.[357] McInnes has conceptualised 'Post-Traumatic Stress Response' similarly: as women's rational responses to men's violence.[358]

A key concept underpinning these analyses is that justifiable distress is not a disease. In the case of PMS, Zita argues that speaking of 'symptoms' detracts from the fact that a woman 'might be furious with someone, and justifiably so'.[359] Indeed, Chrisler and Caplan report that when direct-to-consumer advertisements for Sarafem began to air, many women were aghast that their 'daily frustrations and irritations of life' were being 'portrayed as symptoms of a psychiatric disorder'.[360] Browne's critique of the *DSM-5* is relevant here, for she argues that the manual medicalises 'normal/natural responses to experiences'.[361] We might then say that the manual is complicit in the medicalisation of mental distress.

When it comes to the medicalisation of *women's* mental distress, an oft-raised issue in feminist analyses is that of language. For PMS, author and academic Anne E. Figert notes that the word 'syndrome' implies the existence of 'an underlying disease process in women's bodies'.[362] Social Anxiety *Disorder* arguably has the same implication. Labelling something thus, as Chrisler and Caplan observe, means that 'it is taken more seriously and seen as needing medical attention'.[363] But as social work scholar Susan Gair states, defining experiences as disorders has another effect. For instance, the 'sick label' inherent in the PPD diagnosis dismisses 'the impossible workload, the loss of uninterrupted sleep, and the overwhelming responsibility of motherhood'.[364] Likewise, feminist activist Sophie Laws and colleagues tell us that the PMDD label cleaves women from 'the unfair burdens and circumstances' of their lives.[365] Labelling women's mental distress as a medical issue therefore places 'a biological or medical label on their rebellion or discontent, and thereby dismisses it'.[366] Not only does medicalisation veil the role of environmental factors in women's mental distress,[367] but it posits that the pathology is individual[368] as opposed to being 'a collective social issue'.[369]

When work *does* attempt to examine external factors, there can sometimes still be shortcomings. Mauthner tells us that, in the case of PPD, the analysis often 'fails to go beyond the level of the individual to address the wider sociopolitical and ideological context and structures in which these mothers' experiences are embedded'.[370] Ussher picks up on a similar tendency in the PMS literature, where the phenomenon is presented as a 'disorder affecting an individual woman [...] on whom [...] psychosocial factors impact and produce symptomatology'.[371] The sinister ramification of this constricted view is that the root causes of women's mental distress—'abusive relationships, stressful life circumstances, poverty, trauma, and harassment'[372]—are allowed to continue, unchallenged.[373] Browne's discussion of abuse exemplifies this point. Diagnosing the victim with a 'disorder' ultimately blames her and diverts attention away from the abuser.[374] Further to Browne's example, *medicating* a victim of abuse not only fails to address the cause of her mental distress,[375] but could well facilitate its continuation.[376] Browne draws parallels with such situations and using drugs and alcohol 'as self-medication in order to tolerate otherwise intolerable situations'.[377]

If we are to be critical of medicalising, and medicating, mental distress, it is pertinent to ask *how* the underlying causes can be addressed without endorsing the individual pathology model and turning a blind eye to context. The work of sexologist Leonore Tiefer, whose remit is female sexual problems, acts as a blueprint in this endeavour. Tiefer's 'New View Campaign' challenges 'the medicalization of sex':[378] that is, it challenges the 'framework that reduces sexual problems to disorders of physiological function', wherein their 'socio-cultural, political, psychological, social or relational bases' are ignored.[379]

Echoing critics of biological psychiatry and biological reductionism, Tiefer disputes the dominant framing of FSD—that is, 'strictly physiological'—which focuses on 'fixing the body' with pharmaceuticals.[380] Instead, Tiefer proposes that female sexual problems are contingent on context and may arise from a number of cultural, political, and social factors which specifically affect women. Writing on Tiefer's work, academic and author Katherine Angel cites the following examples: '[L]ack of communication between partners; exhaustion due to inequalities in child-rearing and housework; anxieties about body image; violence from sexual partners; and misunderstandings of female anatomy'.[381]

In the spirit of Tiefer's approach, in this book I am critical of what I see as psychiatry's biological reductionism regarding SAD in women. In order to provide a corrective to dominant narratives on this diagnosis, my focus is on the cultural, social, and political contributors which specifically affect women. In concluding this section, I will cite the Boston Women's Health Collective's stance regarding the medicalisation of women's problems. They state that 'the cure for PMS may lie in resocialization and societal change, not medicine'.[382] Analogously, the cure for women's social anxiety may not lie in psychiatry, but may instead lie in collective resistance to, and resulting change in, societal attitudes regarding what constitutes acceptable behaviours for women.

Holistic Perspective

Throughout this chapter, I have been critical of the idea that mental distress—and, in the chapter's latter half, *women's* mental distress especially—arises from innate, individual, biological pathology. It might be tempting to extrapolate this critique and construe that I am denying the effect of biological factors altogether. While such denial could be seen as 'understandable as a reaction to biological reductionism',[383] as Ussher notes in the case of PMS, it reveals a problem inherent in a social constructionist approach: the body and its effects are not irrelevant. In acknowledging this, I take a stance akin to that of psychologist and midwife Elizabeth Mollard in her analysis of PPD. This viewpoint examines the cultural, biological, psychological, economic, and social aspects of a woman's life, as well as her experiences[384]—something that this book will achieve by exploring women's stories through in-depth interviews.

Adopting this position is necessary to encapsulate the many levels on which women's mental distress occurs. Likewise, writing of PMS, Ussher cites bodily, social, and psychological levels which cannot be disentangled.[385] Mollard espouses an idea akin to this in proposing that women cannot be divided up into parts, and she emphasises the link between the biological and the psychological.[386] That is, the 'way an individual thinks and experiences the world is related to one's biological makeup'.[387] The most obvious, and perhaps most simple, way to relate this to SAD would be to consider its physical manifestations, such as blushing or hand tremor.[388] Concern that others notice these 'symptoms' can then become the focal point of the social anxiety,[389] potentially exacerbating them and, in turn, exacerbating the social anxiety itself. This is but one example of how the intertwinement of the biological with the psychological might play out in social anxiety. Indeed, how this interplay is experienced by the women in my sample will be unpacked, by deploying the holistic perspective outlined above, in the chapters that follow.

Notes

1. Roy Porter, *The Greatest Benefit to Mankind: A Medical History of Humanity* (London: Fontana Press, 1999), p. 493.
2. Michel Foucault, *History of Madness*, ed. by Jean Khalfa; trans. Jonathan Murphy and Jean Khalfa (London, Routledge, 2006), p. 25.
3. Michel Foucault, *Madness and Civilization: A History of Insanity in the Age of Reason* [based on an abridged version of *Folie et Déraison: Histoire de la Folie à L'âge Classique*] trans. Richard Howard (London and New York: Routledge, 2001[1961]), p. xii.
4. Foucault, *History of Madness*, p. 47.
5. Ibid., p. 66.
6. Franz G. Alexander and Sheldon T. Selesnick, *A History of Psychiatry: An Evaluation of Psychiatric Thought and Practice from Prehistoric Times to the Present* (London: George Allen and Unwin, 1967), cited in Oliver Josef Dumolo Ralley, 'The Rise of Anti-psychiatry: A Historical Review', *History of Medicine Online*, 2012 http://www.priory.com/history_of_medicine/Anti-Psychiatry.htm [accessed 10 April 2019].
7. Foucault, *History of Madness*, p. 372.
8. Ronald David Laing, *The Divided Self: An Existential Study in Sanity and Madness* (London: Tavistock Publications Ltd., 1965), p. 12.
9. Porter, *The Greatest Benefit to Mankind*, p. 509.
10. Alexander and Selesnick, *A History of Psychiatry*, cited in Ralley, 'The Rise of Anti-psychiatry'.
11. Isaac Baker Brown, *On the Curability of Certain Forms of Insanity, Epilepsy, Catalepsy, and Hysteria in Females* (Dyke: Harwicke, 1866).
12. Lisa Appignanesi, *Mad, Bad and Sad: A History of Women and the Mind Doctors from 1800 to the Present* (London: Virago, 2008), p. 119.
13. Elaine Showalter, *The Female Malady: Women, Madness, and English Culture* (New York: Pantheon, 1985), pp. 55–56.
14. Helen King, 'Once Upon a Text: Hysteria from Hippocrates', in *Hysteria Beyond Freud*, ed. by Sander L. Gilman, Helen King, Roy Porter, G. S. Rousseau, and Elaine Showalter (Berkeley and Los Angeles: University of California Press, 1993), 3–90.

15. Edward Jorden, 'A Briefe Discourse of a Disease Called the Suffocation of the Mother', (1603) https://quod.lib.umich.edu/e/eebo2/A04663.0001.001?view=toc [accessed 3 January 2021].
16. Laurinda S. Dixon, *Perilous Chastity: Women and Illness in Pre-enlightenment Art and Medicine* (Ithaca and London: Cornell University Press, 1995), pp. 19–20.
17. Gilman et al., *Hysteria Beyond Freud*, p. 118.
18. American Psychiatric Association [APA], *Diagnostic and Statistical Manual of Mental Disorders*, 4*th* edn [*DSM-IV*] (Washington, DC: American Psychiatric Association Publishing, 2000).
19. Jane M. Ussher and Janette Perz, 'PMS as a Gendered Illness Linked to the Construction and Relational Experience of Hetero-femininity', *Sex Roles*, 68 (2013), 132–50 https://doi.org/10.1007/s11199-011-9977-5 p. 132.
20. Showalter, *The Female Malady*.
21. Ibid., pp. 52–53.
22. Ibid.
23. Ibid., p. 51.
24. Ibid., p. 18.
25. Ibid.
26. Ibid., p. 54.
27. Ibid., p. 78.
28. Baker Brown, *On the Curability of Certain Forms of Insanity*.
    Porter, *The Greatest Benefit to Mankind*, p. 520.
29. Porter, *The Greatest Benefit to Mankind*, cited in Ralley, 'The Rise of Anti-psychiatry'.
30. Gerald Grob, *Mental Illness and American Society, 1875–1940* (Princeton: Princeton University Press, 1983), cited in Carl I. Cohen, 'The Biomedicalization of Psychiatry: A Critical Overview', *Community Mental Health Journal*, 29.6 (1993), 509–21 https://doi.org/10.1007/BF00754260 p. 515.
31. Andrew Scull, 'Deinstitutionalization: Cycles of Despair', *Journal of Mind and Behavior*, 11.3–4 (1990), 301–12 https://www.jstor.org/stable/43854093 [accessed 4 January 2021].
32. National Institute for Health and Care Excellence [NICE] *Social Anxiety Disorder: Recognition, Assessment and Treatment* (2013) https://www.nice.org.uk/guidance/cg159 [accessed 11 June 2019].
33. Cohen, 'The Biomedicalization of Psychiatry', p. 515.
34. Ibid.
35. Joel Kovel, 'The American Mental Health Industry', in *Critical Psychiatry*, ed. by David Ingleby (New York: Pantheon, 1980), 72–101.
36. Foucault, *Madness and Civilization*, pp. 234–64.

37. Thierry Haustgen, 'À Propos du Centenaire de la Psychasthénie (1903): Les Troubles Obsessionnels-Compulsifs dans la Psychiatrie Française: Revue Historique', *Annales Médico-psychologiques, Revue Psychiatrique*, 162.6 (2004), 427–40 https://doi.org/10.1016/j.amp.2003.09.012
38. Porter, *The Greatest Benefit to Mankind*, p. 520.
39. Caroline King and Lakshmi N. P. Voruganti, 'What's in a Name? The Evolution of the Nomenclature of Antipsychotic Drugs', *Journal of Psychiatry and Neuroscience*, 27.3 (2002), 168–75 https://pubmed.ncbi.nlm.nih.gov/12066446/ [accessed 4 January 2021].
40. David Healy, 'The Antidepressant Drama', in *The Treatment of Depression: Bridging the 21st Century*, ed. by Myrna Weissman (Washington: American Psychiatric Publishing Inc., 2001), 10–11.
41. Hugh J. Parry, 'Use of Psychotropic Drugs by US Adults', *Public Health Reports*, 83.10 (1968), 799–810 https://doi.org/10.2307/4593420
Hugh J. Parry, Mitchell B. Balter, Glen D. Mellinger, Ira H. Cisin, and Dean I. Manheimer, 'National Patterns of Psychotherapeutic Drug Use', *Archives of General Psychiatry*, 28.6 (1973), 769–38 https://doi.org/10.1001/archpsyc.1973.01750360007002
Mitchell B. Balter, Jerome Levine, and Dean I. Manheimer, 'Cross-National Study of the Extent of Anti-anxiety/Sedative Drug Use', *New England Journal of Medicine*, 290 (1974), 769–74 https://doi.org/10.1056/NEJM197404042901404
All cited in Jonathan M. Metzl, '"Mother's Little Helper": The Crisis of Psychoanalysis and the Miltown Resolution', *Gender and History*, 15.2 (2003), 228–55 https://doi.org/10.1111/1468-0424.00300 p. 228.
42. Porter, *The Greatest Benefit to Mankind*, cited in Ralley, 'The Rise of Anti-psychiatry'.
43. Porter, *The Greatest Benefit to Mankind*, p. 521.
44. Cohen, 'The Biomedicalization of Psychiatry', p. 516.
45. Alvin Pam, 'A Critique of the Scientific Status of Biological Psychiatry: Part II: Errors in Conception', *Acta Psychiatrica Scandinavica*, 82.S362 (1990), 1–35 https://doi.org/10.1111/j.1600-0447.1990.tb06868.x p. 28.
46. Brett J. Deacon, 'The Biomedical Model of Mental Disorder: A Critical Analysis of its Validity, Utility, and Effects on Psychotherapy Research', *Clinical Psychology Review*, 33.7 (2013), 846–61 https://doi.org/10.1016/j.cpr.2012.09.007
47. Scott A. Dowling, 'George Engel, M.D. (1913–1999)', *The American Journal of Psychiatry*, 162.11 (2005), 2039 https://doi.org/10.1176/appi.ajp.162.11.2039
48. George L. Engel, 'The Need for a New Medical Model: A Challenge for Biomedicine', *Science*, 196.4286 (1977), 129–36 https://doi.org/10.1126/science.847460 p. 129.

49. Alan F. Schatzberg, 'Presidential Address', *The American Journal of Psychiatry*, 167.10 (2010), 1162–65 https://doi.org/10.1176/appi.ajp.2009.166.10.1105 [accessed 4 January 2021] p. 1163.
50. Deacon, 'The Biomedical Model of Mental Disorder', p. 848.
51. Cohen, 'The Biomedicalization of Psychiatry', p. 512.
52. Phil Brown, 'Diagnostic Conflict and Contradiction in Psychiatry', *Journal of Health and Social Behavior*, 28.1 (1987), 37–50 https://doi.org/10.2307/2137139 cited in Cohen, 'The Biomedicalization of Psychiatry', p. 518.
53. Paula J. Caplan, 'The Great "Crazy" Cover-up and Its Human Costs', *Mad in America* (n.d.) https://www.madinamerica.com/wp-content/uploads/2014/02/The-Great-_Crazy_Coverup.pdf [accessed 6 November 2022] p. 2.
54. Paula J. Caplan and Lisa Cosgrove, 'Is this Really Necessary?' in *Bias in Psychiatric Diagnosis*, ed. by Paula J. Caplan and Lisa Cosgrove (Northvale: Jason Aronson Inc., 2004), xix–xxxii, p. xx.
55. Thomas S. Szasz, *The Myth of Mental Illness: Foundations of a Theory of Personal Conduct* (New York: Harper and Row, 1974).
56. Cohen, 'The Biomedicalization of Psychiatry', p. 509.
57. Engel, 'The Need for a New Medical Model', cited in Deacon, 'The Biomedical Model of Mental Disorder', p. 847.
58. Cohen, 'The Biomedicalization of Psychiatry', pp. 509–10.
59. Bruce. G. Charlton, 'A Critique of Biological Psychiatry', *Psychological Medicine*, 20.1 (1990), 3–6 https://doi.org/10.1017/s0033291700013179 p. 5.
60. Ibid.
61. Steven P. R. Rose, *Molecules and Minds* (Milton Keynes: Open University Press, 1987), cited in Charlton, 'A Critique of Biological Psychiatry', p. 5.
62. Richard Rorty, *Consequences of Pragmatism* (Brighton: Harvester, 1982), cited in Charlton, 'A Critique of Biological Psychiatry', p. 5.
63. Rose, *Molecules and Minds.*
64. Charlton, 'A Critique of Biological Psychiatry', p. 5.
65. Engel, 'The Need for a New Medical Model', p. 130.
66. Cohen, 'The Biomedicalization of Psychiatry', p. 512.
67. Milena Büchs, 'Social Pathology', *The Blackwell Encyclopedia of Sociology* (2007) https://doi.org/10.1002/9781405165518.wbeoss173
68. Cohen, 'The Biomedicalization of Psychiatry', p. 517.
69. Angela K. Thachuk, 'Stigma and the Politics of Biomedical Models of Mental Illness', *International Journal of Feminist Approaches to Bioethics*, 4.1 (2011), 140–63 https://doi.org/10.3138/ijfab.4.1.140 p. 144.
70. Cohen, 'The Biomedicalization of Psychiatry', p. 517.
71. Ibid.

72. Conrad, 'On the Medicalization of Deviance and Social Control'.
73. Michel Foucault, *Ethics: Subjectivity and Truth: Essential Works of Michel Foucault 1954–1984, Vol. 1*, ed. by Paul Rabinow, trans. Robert Hurley and others (New York: New York Press, 1997), p. 313.
74. Cohen, 'The Biomedicalization of Psychiatry', p. 511.
75. Pam, 'A Critique of the Scientific Status of Biological Psychiatry', p. 24.
76. Cohen, 'The Biomedicalization of Psychiatry', p. 511.
77. Szasz, *The Myth of Mental Illness*, p. 182.
78. Paula J. Caplan, *When Jonny and Jane Come Marching Home: How all of Us Can Help Veterans* (Hanover, NH: Scribl, 2019), p. 30.
79. Ibid., p. 23.
80. Presidential Lecture, Society of Biological Psychiatry, *Clinical Psychiatry News*, 17.7 (July 1989), cited in Cohen, 'The Biomedicalization of Psychiatry', p. 513.
81. Peter D. Kramer, *Listening to Prozac* (London: Fourth Estate, 1994), p. xiii.
82. Stanley W. Jackson, *Melancholia and Depression: From Hippocratic Times to Modern Times* (New Haven, CT: Yale University Press, 1986), cited in Michelle N. Lafrance, 'A Bitter Pill: A Discursive Analysis of Women's Medicalized Accounts of Depression', *Journal of Health Psychology*, 12.1 (2007), 127–40 https://doi.org/10.1177/1359105307071746
83. Paula Gardner, 'Distorted Packaging: Marketing Depression as Illness, Drugs as Cure', *Journal of Medical Humanities*, 24.1–2 (2003), 105–30 https://doi.org/10.1023/A:1021314017235 cited in Lafrance, 'A Bitter Pill', p. 128.
84. Christopher M. France, Paul H. Lysaker, and Ryan P. Robinson, 'The "Chemical Imbalance" Explanation for Depression: Origins, Lay Endorsement, and Clinical Implications', *Professional Psychology: Research and Practice*, 38.4 (2007), 411–20 https://doi.org/10.1037/0735-7028.38.4.411
85. Jeffrey R. Lacasse and Jonathan Leo, 'Serotonin and Depression: A Disconnect between the Advertisements and the Scientific Literature', *PLoS Medicine*, 2.12 e192 (2005), 1211–16 https://doi.org/10.1371/journal.pmed.0020392 cited in Deacon, 'The Biomedical Model of Mental Disorder', p. 849.
86. Thachuk, 'Stigma and the Politics of Biomedical Models', p. 146.
87. Bernice A. Pescosolido, Jack K. Martin, Scott Long, Tait R. Medina, Jo C. Phelan, and Bruce G. Link, 'A Disease Like any Other? A Decade of Change in Public Reactions to Schizophrenia, Depression, and Alcohol Dependence', *The American Journal of Psychiatry*, 167 (2010), 1321–30 https://doi.org/10.1176/appi.ajp.2010.09121743 p. 1327.

88. Matthias C. Angermeyer and Herbert Matschinger, 'Labeling – Stereotype – Discrimination: An Investigation of the Stigma Process', *Social Psychiatry and Psychiatric Epidemiology*, 40.5 (2005), 391–95 https://doi.org/10.1007/s00127-005-0903-4
D. J. Hill and R. M. Bale, *Measuring Beliefs about where Psychological Distress Originates and Who Is Responsible for its Alleviation* (New York: Academic Press, 1981).
Sheila Mehta and Amerigo Farina, 'Is Being "Sick" Really Better? Effect of the Disease View of Mental Disorder on Stigma', *Journal of Social and Clinical Psychology*, 16.4 (1997), 405–19 https://doi.org/10.1521/jscp.1997.16.4.405
All cited in Brett J. Deacon and Grayson L. Baird, 'The Chemical Imbalance Explanation of Depression: Reducing Blame at What Cost?', *Journal of Social and Clinical Psychology*, 28.4 (2009), 415–35 https://doi.org/10.1521/jscp.2009.28.4.415 pp. 430–31.
89. Ibid.
90. Ibid.
91. Talcott Parsons, *The Social System* (New York and Toronto: The Free Press, 1964), p. 314.
92. Ibid., p. 437.
93. Ibid., p. 440.
94. Angermeyer and Matschinger, 'Labeling – Stereotype – Discrimination'.
Hill and Bale, *Measuring Beliefs about where Psychological Distress Originates.*
Mehta and Farina, 'Is Being "Sick" Really Better?'
All cited in Deacon and Baird, 'The Chemical Imbalance Explanation of Depression', pp. 430–31.
95. Deacon and Baird, 'The Chemical Imbalance Explanation of Depression', pp. 430–31.
96. Donald J. Kiesler, *Beyond the Disease Model of Mental Disorders* (Westport, CT: Praeger, 2000).
97. Hyman at the 1999 White House Conference on Mental Health, quoted in George W. Albee and Justin M. Joffe, 'Mental illness Is NOT an "Illness Like any Other"', *The Journal of Primary Prevention*, 24 (2004), 419–36 https://doi.org/10.1023/B:JOPP.0000024799.04666.8b cited in Deacon, 'The Biomedical Model of Mental Disorder', pp. 851–52.
98. Marcia Angell, 'The Illusions of Psychiatry', *The New York Times Review of Books* (2011) http://www.nybooks.com/articles/archives/2011/jul/14/illusions-of-psychiatry/ [accessed 18 February 2012].
Marcia Angell, 'The Epidemic of Mental illness: Why?', *The New York Times Review of Books* (2011) http://www.nybooks.com/articles/archives/2011/jun/23/epidemic-mental-illness-why/ [accessed 18 February 2012].

Sharon Begley, 'The Depressing News about Antidepressants', *Newsweek* (2010) http://www.thedailybeast.com/newsweek/2010/01/28/the-depressing-news-about-antidepressants.html [accessed 18 February 2012].
Alix Spiegel, *When It Comes to Depression, Serotonin Isn't the Whole Story* (2012) http://www.npr.org/blogs/health/2012/01/23/145525853/when-it-comes-to-depression-serotonin-isnt-the-whole-story [accessed 18 February 2012].
Lesley Stahl, 'Treating Depression: Is there a Placebo Effect?' *60 Minutes* (2012) http://www.cbsnews.com/830118560_162-57380893/treating-depression-is-there-a-placebo-effect/ [accessed 6 March 2012].
All cited in Deacon, 'The Biomedical Model of Mental Disorder', p. 847.

99. Thomas R. Insel, *Mental Illness Defined as Disruption in Neural Circuits* (2011) http://www.nimh.nih.gov/about/director/2011/mental-illness-defined-as-disruption-in-neural-circuits.shtml [accessed 18 February 2012].
Dr Joseph Coyle, quoted in Spiegel, *When it Comes to Depression*, cited in Deacon, 'The Biomedical Model of Mental Disorder', p. 852.
Ronald W. Pies, 'Psychiatry's New Brain-Mind and the Legend of the "Chemical Imbalance"', *Psychiatric News* (2011) http://www.psychiatrictimes.com/blog/couchincrisis/content/article/10168/1902106 [accessed 18 February 2012].
All cited in Deacon, 'The Biomedical Model of Mental Disorder', p. 852.
100. Appignanesi, *Mad, Bad and Sad*, p. 4.
101. Jane M. Ussher, *Women's Madness: Misogyny or Mental Illness?* (London: Harvester Wheatsheaf, 1991), p. 217.
102. Pam, 'A Critique of the Scientific Status of Biological Psychiatry', p. 20.
103. Appignanesi, *Mad, Bad and Sad*, p. 4.
104. World Health Organisation, *Mental Health Global Action Plan: Close the Gap, Dare To Care* (2002) http://www.who.int/mental_health/media/en/265.pdf [accessed 18 February 2005], cited in Philip Thomas, Patrick Bracken, Paul Cutler, Robert Hayward, Rufus May, and Salma Yasmeen, 'Challenging the Globalisation of Biomedical Psychiatry', *Journal of Public Mental Health*, 4.3 (2005), 23–32 https://doi.org/10.1108/17465729200500021 p. 25.
105. Deacon, 'The Biomedical Model of Mental Disorder', p. 847.
106. Pam, 'A Critique of the Scientific Status of Biological Psychiatry', pp. 12–13, 18.
107. Sami Timimi, 'No More Psychiatric Labels: Why Formal Psychiatric Diagnostic Systems Should Be Abolished', *International Journal of Clinical and Health Psychology*, 14.3 (2014), 208–15 https://doi.org/10.1016/j.ijchp.2014.03.004 p. 209.

108. The Association of the British Pharmaceutical Industry, *Did You Know?: Facts and Figures about the Pharmaceutical Industry in the UK – Second edn* (2011) http://www.abpi.org.uk/our-work/library/industry/Documents/Did%20you%20know_Jan11.pdf [accessed 13 March 2019].
109. Peter Gøtzsche, *Deadly Medicines and Organised Crime: How Big Pharma Has Corrupted Healthcare* (New York: Radcliffe, 2013).
110. Blair T. Johnson and Irving Kirsch, 'Do Antidepressants Work? Statistical Significance versus Clinical Benefits', *Significance*, 5.2 (2008), 54–58 https://doi.org/10.1111/j.1740-9713.2008.00286.x p. 54.
111. Gareth Iacobucci, 'NHS Prescribed Record Number of Antidepressants Last Year', *British Medical Journal*, 364.1508 (2019) https://doi.org/10.1136/bmj.l1508
112. S. Pilling, E. Mayo-Wilson, I. Mavranezouli, K. Kew, C. Taylor, and D. M. Clark (Guideline Development Group), 'Recognition, Assessment and Treatment of Social Anxiety Disorder: Summary of NICE Guidance', *British Medical Journal (Clinical Research Ed.)*, 346.f2541 (2013) https://doi.org/10.1136/bmj.f2541
113. Mind, *We Need To Talk: Getting the Right Therapy at the Right Time* (n.d.) https://www.mind.org.uk/media/280583/We-Need-to-Talk-getting-the-right-therapy-at-the-right-time.pdf [accessed 10 June 2019].
114. Ibid.
115. NHS England, *Adult Improving Access to Psychological Therapies Programme* (n.d.) https://www.england.nhs.uk/mental-health/adults/iapt/ [accessed 7 January 2021].
116. Mind, *We Need To Talk*.
117. NHS England, *Adult Improving Access to Psychological Therapies Programme*.
118. British Medical Association [BMA], *Pressure Points in the NHS* (2021) https://www.bma.org.uk/advice-and-support/nhs-delivery-and-workforce/pressures/pressure-points-in-the-nhs [accessed 22 February 2021]. NHS England, *Consultant-led Referral to Treatment Waiting Times Data 2020-21* (2020) https://www.england.nhs.uk/statistics/statistical-work-areas/rtt-waiting-times/rtt-data-2020-21/ [accessed 22 February 2021], cited in Shaun Griffin, 'Covid-19: Waiting Times in England Reach Record Highs', *British Medical Journal* (2020) 370.m3557, 1 https://doi.org/10.1136/bmj.m3557
119. Mind, *Mind Warns of 'Second Pandemic' as it Reveals More People in Mental Health Crisis than ever Recorded and Helpline Calls Soar* (2020) https://www.mind.org.uk/news-campaigns/news/mind-warns-of-second-pandemic-as-it-reveals-more-people-in-mental-health-crisis-than-ever-recorded-and-helpline-calls-soar/ [accessed 22 February 2021].

120. Julia Hyde, Michael Calnan, Lindsay Prior, Glyn Lewis, David Kessler, and Deborah Sharp, 'A Qualitative Study Exploring how GPs Decide To Prescribe Antidepressants', *British Journal of General Practice*, 55.519 (2005), 755–62 https://www.ncbi.nlm.nih.gov/pmc/articles/PMC1562347/ [accessed 25 September 2020] pp. 759–60.
Royal Pharmaceutical Society, 'Most GPs are Over-prescribing Antidepressants', *The Pharmaceutical Journal Online*, 272.7293 (2004), 407 https://www.pharmaceutical-journal.com/pj-online-news-most-gps-are-over-prescribing-antidepressants/20011591.article?firstPass=false [accessed 10 June 2019].
Emily Wooster on behalf of the We Need To Talk campaign, *While We are Waiting: Experiences of Waiting for and Receiving Psychological Therapies on the NHS* (2019) https://www.mentalhealth.org.uk/publications/while-we-are-waiting [accessed 10 June 2019] p. 8.
121. Anvishka Patel, *Government Must Stop Cutting Funding for 'Deteriorating' Public Health Services* (2019) http://www.pulsetoday.co.uk/news/hot-topics/public-health-cuts/government-must-stop-cutting-funding-for-deteriorating-public-health-services/20038466.article [accessed 10 June 2019].
122. British Medical Association, *Prioritising Prevention for Population Health* (2019) https://www.bma.org.uk/collective-voice/policy-and-research/public-and-population-health/prioritising-prevention-for-population-health [accessed 7 January 2021].
Trade Union Congress, *Breaking Point: The Crisis in Mental Health Funding* (2018) https://www.tuc.org.uk/sites/default/files/Mentalhealthfundingreport2_0.pdf [accessed 10 June 2019].
123. Allan V. Horwitz, *Creating Mental Illness* (London: University of Chicago Press, 2002), cited in Olivia Goldhill, *30 Years After Prozac Arrived, We Still Buy the Lie that Chemical Imbalances Cause Depression* (2019) https://qz.com/1162154/30-years-after-prozac-arrived-we-still-buy-the-lie-that-chemical-imbalances-cause-depression/ [accessed 10 June 2019].
124. Cohen, 'The Biomedicalization of Psychiatry', p. 517.
125. Iacobucci, 'NHS Prescribed Record Number of Antidepressants'.
126. In brief, these include Generalised Anxiety Disorder (GAD), Depressive Episode (mild, moderate or severe), Phobias, Obsessive-compulsive Disorder, and Panic Disorder. For further detail, see P. McManus, R. Bebbington, R. Jenkins, and T. Brugha (eds.), *Mental Health and Wellbeing in England: Adult Psychiatric Morbidity Survey 2014* (Leeds: NHS Digital, 2016) https://assets.publishing.service.gov.uk/government/uploads/system/uploads/attachment_data/file/556596/apms-2014-full-rpt.pdf [accessed 28 April 2023] pp. 389–90.

127. One adult in six adults was found to have a (CMD); one in five women and one in eight men.
Ibid., p. 8.
128. James Banks and Xiaowei Xu, 'The Mental Health Effects of the First Two Months of Lockdown and Social Distancing During the Covid-19 Pandemic in the UK', Institute of Fiscal Studies Working Paper W20/16 (2020) https://doi.org/10.1920/wp.ifs.2020.1620
129. Michael E. Thase, 'Do Antidepressants really Work? A Clinicians' Guide to Evaluating the Evidence', *Current Psychiatry Reports*, 10.6 (2008) 487–94 https://doi.org/10.1007/s11920-008-0078-2
Lisa Bero, Fieke Oostvogel, Peter Bacchetti, and Kirby Lee, 'Factors Associated with Findings of Published Trials of Drug-Drug Comparisons: Why Some Statins Appear More Efficacious than Others', *PLoS Medicine*, 4.6 (2007) e184 https://doi.org/10.1371/journal.pmed.0040184 cited in Ben Goldacre, *Bad Pharma* (London: Fourth Estate, 2012), p. 2.
130. Goldacre, *Bad Pharma*, p. xi.
131. Ibid., p. 171.
132. Ibid., pp. 216–17.
133. Ibid., pp. 176, 180–87, 191–93.
134. Ibid., pp. 12, 407.
135. Ibid.
136. Irving Kirsch, 'Antidepressants and the Placebo Effect', *ZeitschriftfürPsychologie*, 222.3 (2014), 128–34 https://doi.org/10.1027/2151-2604/a000176 p. 128.
137. Ibid.
138. Johnson and Kirsch, 'Do Antidepressants Work?', p. 56.
139. Sometimes euphemistically termed 'discontinuation syndrome'.
140. Kirsch, 'Antidepressants and the Placebo Effect', p. 132.
141. Paul W. Andrews, J. Anderson Thomson, Jr., Ananda Amstadter, and Michael C. Neale, 'Primum Non Nocere: An Evolutionary Analysis of whether Antidepressants Do More Harm than Good' [Review], *Frontiers in Psychology*, 3.117 (2012) https://doi.org/10.3389/fpsyg.2012.00117
M. A. Babyak, J. A. Blumenthal, S. Herman, P. Khatri, P. M. Doraiswamy, K. A. Moore, and K. R. Krishnan, 'Exercise Treatment for Major Depression: Maintenance of Therapeutic Benefit at 10 Months', *Psychosomatic Medicine*, 62 (2000), 633–38 https://doi.org/10.1097/00006842-200009000-00006
Keith S. Dobson, Steven D. Hollon, Sona Dimidjian, Karen B. Schmaling, Robert J. Kohlenberg, Robert Gallop, Shireen L. Rizvi, Jackie K. Gollan, David L. Dunner, and Neil S. Jacobson, 'Randomized Trial of Behavioral Activation, Cognitive Therapy, and Antidepressant Medication in the Prevention of Relapse and Recurrence in Major Depression', *Journal of*

Consulting and Clinical Psychology, 76.3 (2008), 468–77 https://doi.org/10.1037/0022-006X.76.3.468
All cited in Kirsch, 'Antidepressants and the Placebo Effect', p. 132.
142. Kirsch, 'Antidepressants and the Placebo Effect', p. 128.
143. Deacon, 'The Biomedical Model of Mental Disorder', p. 846.
144. Kenneth S. Kendler and Kenneth F. Schaffner, 'The Dopamine Hypothesis of Schizophrenia: An Historical and Philosophical Analysis', *Philosophy in Psychiatry and Psychology*, 18.1 (2011), 41–63 https://doi.org/10.1353/ppp.2011.0005
Irving Kirsch, *The Emperor's New Drugs: Exploding the Antidepressant Myth* (New York: Basic Books, 2010).
Lacasse and Leo, 'Serotonin and Depression'.
All cited in Deacon, 'The Biomedical Model of Mental Disorder', p. 852.
145. Philip J. Cowen and Michael Browning. 'What Has Serotonin To Do with Depression?' *World Psychiatry*, 14.2 (2015), 158–60 https://doi.org/10.1002/wps.20229 p. 160.
146. Kirsch, 'Antidepressants and the Placebo Effect', p. 128.
147. Ibid., p. 131.
For further discussion of antidepressants and the placebo effect, see Katie Masters, 'Placebo', *Index of Evidence* (2021) https://www.indexofevidence.org/placebo-effect [accessed 6 April 2023].
148. Appignanesi, *Mad, Bad and Sad*, p. 448.
149. Pam, 'A Critique of the Scientific Status of Biological Psychiatry', p. 11.
150. Ibid., p. 21.
151. Ibid., p. 12.
152. Ibid.
153. David Healy, *Pharmageddon* (Berkeley, California: University of California Press, 2012), p. 35.
154. Joanna Moncrieff, *Is Psychiatry for Sale? An Examination of the Influence of the Pharmaceutical Industry on Academic and Practical Psychiatry*, Maudsley Discussion Paper (London: Institute of Psychiatry, 2003).
155. Barry Brand, quoted in Shankar Vedantam, 'Drug Ads Hyping Anxiety Make Some Uneasy', *Washington Post* (16 July 2001) https://www.washingtonpost.com/archive/politics/2001/07/16/drug-ads-hyping-anxiety-make-some-uneasy/8fe2eea2-b780-48cd-9872-1d3802e83147/ [accessed 7 January 2021].
156. Lane, *Shyness*.
157. Goldacre, *Bad Pharma*, pp. 261–62.
158. Edward O. Laumann, Anthony Paik, and Raymond C. Rosen, 'Sexual Dysfunction in the United States: Prevalence and Predictors', *Journal of the American Medical Association*, 281.6 (1999), 537–44 https://doi.org/10.1001/jama.281.6.537

159. Goldacre, *Bad Pharma*, pp. 261–62.
160. Denise Grady, 'THE NATION: BETTER LOVING THROUGH CHEMISTRY; Sure, We've Got a Pill for That', *New York Times* (1999) https://www.nytimes.com/1999/02/14/weekinreview/the-nation-better-loving-through-chemistry-sure-we-ve-got-a-pill-for-that.html [accessed 11 June 2019], cited in Goldacre, *Bad Pharma*, pp. 261–62.
161. McInnes, 'The Personal Is Political', p. 161.
162. Ibid., p. 160.
163. Goldacre, *Bad Pharma*, p. 123.
164. Pam, 'A Critique of the Scientific Status of Biological Psychiatry', p. 28.
165. Robert Whitaker, *Anatomy of an Epidemic: Magic Bullets, Psychiatric Drugs, and the Astonishing Rise of Mental Illness in America* (New York: Crown, 2010), cited in Deacon, 'The Biomedical Model of Mental Disorder', p. 848.
166. Thomas et al., 'Challenging the Globalisation of Biomedical Psychiatry', p. 23.
167. 1 Boring Old Man, *Not a Toy...* (2012) http://1boringoldman.com/index.php/2012/06/09/not-a-toy/ [accessed 7 January 2021].
Dx Revision Watch, *Three Professional Organization Responses to Third and Final DSM-5 Stakeholder Review* (2012) http://dxrevisionwatch.wordpress.com/2012/06/21/three-professional-organization-responses-to-third-and-final-dsm-5-stakeholder-review [accessed 25 June 2020].
Allen J. Frances and Thomas Widiger, 'Psychiatric Diagnosis: Lessons from the DSM-IV Past and Cautions for the Future', *Annual Review of Clinical Psychology*, 8 (2012), 109–30 https://doi.org/10.1146/annurev-clinpsy-032511-143102
Brent Robbins, *Open Letter to the DSM-5* (n.d) http://www.ipetitions.com/petition/dsm5/ [accessed 4 February 2013].
Brian C. Pilecki, J. W. Clegg, and D. McKay, 'The Influence of Corporate and Political Interests on Models of Illness in the Evolution of the DSM', *European Psychiatry*, 26.3 (2011), 194–200 https://doi.org/10.1016/j.eurpsy.2011.01.005
All cited in Deacon, 'The Biomedical Model of Mental Disorder', p. 852.
168. Peter Schrag, *Mind Control* (New York: Pantheon, 1978), cited in Pam, 'A Critique of the Scientific Status of Biological Psychiatry', p. 28.
169. Appignanesi, *Mad, Bad and Sad*, p. 506.
170. Kramer, *Listening to Prozac*, p. 35.
171. Edward Shorter, *A History of Psychiatry* (New York: John Wiley and Sons, 1997), p. 5.
172. Ibid.
173. Kramer, *Listening to Prozac*, p. 236.

174. Clare Wilson, 'Nobody Can Agree about Antidepressants: Here's What You Need To Know', *New Scientist* (2018) https://www.newscientist.com/article/mg23931980-100-nobody-can-agree-about-antidepressants-heres-what-you-need-to-know/ [accessed 25 September 2020].
175. Kramer, *Listening to Prozac*, p. xv.
176. Ibid., p. 246.
177. Ibid., p. 174.
178. Lane, *Shyness*, p. 9.
179. Kramer, *Listening to Prozac*, p. 237.
180. Ibid., p. 9.
181. Ibid., pp. 10–11.
182. Ibid., p. xvi.
183. Ibid., p. xv.
184. Ibid., p. 162.
185. Ibid., p. xvi.
186. Ibid., p. 143.
187. Ibid., p. 41.
188. Peter Conrad, *The Medicalization of Society: On the Transformation of Human Conditions into Treatable Disorders* (Baltimore, MD: Johns Hopkins University Press, 2008).
189. Kramer, *Listening to Prozac*, p. xv.
190. Ibid., p. 108.
191. Ibid., p. 41.
192. Richard S. Schwartz, 'Mood Brighteners, Affect Tolerance, and the Blues', *Psychiatry*, 54.4 (1991), 397–403 https://doi.org/10.1080/00332747.1991.11024568 p. 401, cited in Kramer, *Listening to Prozac*, p. 254.
193. Ivan Crozier, 'Making up Koro: Multiplicity, Psychiatry, Culture, and Penis-shrinking Anxieties', *Journal of the History of Medicine and Allied Sciences*, 67.1 (2011), 36–70 https://doi.org/10.1093/jhmas/jrr008 p. 65.
194. Ibid., p. 43.
195. Ibid., p. 44.
196. American Psychiatric Association, *Cultural Concepts in DSM-5* (2013) www.psychiatry.org%2FFile%2520Library%2FPsychiatrists%2FPractice%2FDSM%2FAPADSMCultural-Concepts-in-DSM-5.pdf&usg=AOvVaw3_HkTBYb4VAOy0SY3yoZOS [accessed 7 January 2021] p. 1.
197. Ibid.
198. Ibid.
199. Katsuaki Suzuki, Nori Takei, Masayoshi Kawai, Yoshio Minabe, and Norio Mori, 'Is Taijin Kyofusho a Culture-bound Syndrome?' *American*

Journal of Psychiatry, 160.7 (2003), 1358 https://doi.org/10.1176/appi.ajp.160.7.1358 p. 1358.

200. APA, *Cultural Concepts in DSM-5*, p. 1.
201. Charles C. Hughes, 'The Glossary of "Culture-bound Syndromes" in DSM-IV: A Critique', *Transcultural Psychiatry*, 35.3 (1998), 413–21 https://doi.org/10.1177/136346159803500307 p. 420.
202. Hughes, 'The Glossary of "Culture-bound Syndromes"', p. 420.
203. David Ingleby, 'Understanding Mental Illness', in *Critical Psychiatry*, ed. by David Ingleby (New York: Pantheon, 1980), 23–27, cited in Cohen, 'The Biomedicalization of Psychiatry', p. 512.
204. Hughes, 'The Glossary of "Culture-bound Syndromes"', p. 414.
     APA, *Cultural Concepts in DSM-5*, p. 1.
205. Crozier, 'Making Up Koro', pp. 67–68.
206. Ibid.
207. German Berrios and Stephen Morley, 'Koro-like Symptoms in a non-Chinese Subject', *British Journal of Psychiatry*, 145 (1984), 331–34 https://doi.org/10.1192/bjp.145.3.331 p. 333, cited in Crozier, 'Making Up Koro', p. 51.
208. Crozier, 'Making Up Koro', p. 69.
209. Hughes, 'The Glossary of "Culture-bound Syndromes"', p. 420.
210. Ibid.
211. Ibid.
212. Crozier, 'Making Up Koro', pp. 40–41.
213. Richard Dyer, *White* (London: Routledge, 1997).
     bell hooks, *Ain't I a Woman?: Black Women and Feminism* (Boston: South End Press, 1981).
     All cited in Kathy Deliovsky, 'Normative White Femininity: Race, Gender and the Politics of Beauty', *Atlantis: Critical Studies in Gender, Culture and Social Justice*, 33.1 (2008), 49–59 https://journals.msvu.ca/index.php/atlantis/article/view/429 [accessed 30 January 2023] p. 6.
214. Dyer, *White*, cited in Deliovsky, 'Normative White Femininity', pp. 56–57.
215. Sarah Carter, *Capturing Women: The Manipulation of Cultural Imagery in Canada's Prairie West* (Montreal: McGill-Queens University Press, 1997), cited in Deliovsky, 'Normative White Femininity', p. 57.
216. Coventry Patmore, *The Angel in the House*, ed. by Henry Morley (2014 [1891]) https://www.gutenberg.org/files/4099/4099-h/4099-h.htm [accessed 26 September 2020].
217. Virginia Woolf, 'The Professions of Women', in *Virginia Woolf: Selected Essays*, ed. by David Bradshaw (New York: Oxford University Press, 2008), 140–45, p. 141.

218. Laura T. Hamilton, Elizabeth A. Armstrong, J. Lotus Seeley, and Elizabeth M. Armstrong, 'Hegemonic Femininities and Intersectional Domination', *Sociological Theory*, 37.4 (2019), 315–41 https://doi.org/10.1177/0735275119888248
219. Deliovsky, 'Normative White Femininity', p. 57.
220. Sandra L. Bem, 'The Measurement of Psychological Androgyny', *Journal of Consulting and Clinical Psychology*, 42.2 (1974), 155–62 https://doi.org/10.1037/h0036215 p. 156.
221. Ibid.
222. Ibid.
223. Kramer, *Listening to Prozac*, p. 271.
224. Rosalind Gill, 'Postfeminist Media Culture: Elements of a Sensibility', *European Journal of Cultural Studies*, 10.2 (2007), 147–66 https://doi.org/10.1177/1367549407075898 p. 158.
225. Lori B. Girshick, 'The Social Construction of Biological Facts', in *Transgender Voices: Beyond Women and Men*, ed. by Lori B. Girshick (Hanover, New Hampshire: University Press of New England, 2008), 23–50, p. 48.
226. Bem, 'The Measurement of Psychological Androgyny', p. 156.
227. Julia Serano, *Whipping Girl: A Transsexual Woman on Sexism and the Scapegoating of Femininity* (Berkeley: Seal Press, 2007), pp. 284–92.
228. Kramer, *Listening to Prozac*, p. 170.
229. The term 'overly-feminine' is an interesting one—a woman can be feminine, but not *too* feminine—and it speaks to my earlier contention that women are expected to embody contradictory traits simultaneously.
230. Ibid.
231. Ibid., p. 271.
232. Ibid.
233. Metzl, '"Mother's Little Helper"', p. 228.
234. Kramer, *Listening to Prozac*, p. 40.
235. Ibid.
236. Jaqueline Susann, *Valley of the Dolls* (New York: Random House, 1966). Barbara Gordon, *I'm Dancing as Fast as I Can* (New York: Harper and Row, 1979).
    All cited in Metzl, '"Mother's Little Helper"', p. 228.
237. Schwartz, 'Mood Brighteners', cited in Kramer, *Listening to Prozac*, p. 253.
238. McInnes, 'The Political Is Personal', p. 162.
239. Kramer, *Listening to Prozac*, p. 273.
240. McInnes, 'The Political Is Personal', p. 164.
241. Jane M. Ussher, 'Premenstrual Syndrome: Reconciling Disciplinary Divides through the Adoption of a Material-Discursive Epistemological Standpoint', *Annual Review of Sex Research*, 7.1 (1996), 218–51 https://doi.org/10.1080/10532528.1996.10559914 pp. 225, 235.

242. APA, *DSM-5*, p. 171.
243. Kathy Kendall, 'Dangerous Bodies', in *Offenders and Victims: Theory and Policy British Criminology Conference 1991, Selected Papers, Vol. 1*, ed. by David P. Farrington and Sandra Walkate (The British Society of Criminology and the Institute for the Study and Treatment of Delinquency, 1992), p. 48, cited in Kirsten K. Johnson and Mary Anne Kandrack, 'On the Medico-legal Appropriation of Menstrual Discourse: The Syndromization of Women's Experiences', *Resources for Feminist Research*, 24.1/2 (1995), 23–27 [accessed 4 January 2021] p. 23.
244. Johnson and Kandrack, 'On the Medico-legal Appropriation of Menstrual Discourse', p. 23.
245. Sophie Laws, *Issues of Blood: The Politics of Menstruation* (London: MacMillan, 1991).
Mary Brown Parlee, 'The Social Construction of PMS: A Case Study of Scientific Discourse as Cultural Contestation', *The Good Body: Asceticism in Contemporary Culture* conference (Institute for the Medical Humanities, Texas University, Galveston, 1991).
246. Esther Rome, 'Premenstrual Syndrome (PMS) Examined through a Feminist Lens', *Health Care for Women International*, 7.1–2 (1986), 145–51 https://doi.org/10.1080/07399338609515729 p. 145.
247. World Health Organization [WHO] 'Social Phobias', *International Classification of Diseases*, 10th edn [*ICD-10*] (2016) https://icd.who.int/browse10/2016/en#/F40.1 [accessed 25 September 2020].
248. Lynn Payer, *Medicine and Culture* (New York: Henry Holt and Company, 1988).
P. Sedgewick, *Psychopolitics* (London: Pluto Press, 1987).
All cited in Ussher, 'Premenstrual Syndrome: Reconciling Disciplinary Divides', p. 228.
249. Ussher, 'Premenstrual Syndrome: Reconciling Disciplinary Divides', p. 228.
250. Payer, *Medicine and Culture*.
Sedgewick, *Psychopolitics*.
All cited in Ussher, 'Premenstrual Syndrome: Reconciling Disciplinary Divides', p. 228.
251. Joan C. Chrisler and Ingrid Johnston-Robledo, 'Raging Hormones?: Feminist Perspectives on Premenstrual Syndrome and Postpartum Depression', in *Rethinking Mental Health and Disorder: Feminist Perspectives*, ed. by Mary Ballou and Laura S. Brown (New York: Guilford Press, 2002), 174–97, cited in Jane M. Ussher, 'Diagnosing Difficult Women and Pathologising Femininity: Gender Bias in Psychiatric Nosology', *Feminism and Psychology*, 23.1 (2013), 63–69 https://doi.org/10.1177/0959353512467968 p. 66.

Tamara Kayali Browne, 'Is Premenstrual Dysphoric Disorder Really a Disorder?' *Journal of Bioethical Inquiry*, 12.2 (2015), 313–30 https://doi.org/10.1007/s11673-014-9567-7
Thomas M. Johnson, 'Premenstrual Syndrome as a Western Culture-specific Disorder', *Culture, Medicine and Psychiatry*, 11.3 (1987), 337–56 https://doi.org/10.1007/BF00048518
Joan C. Chrisler, 'PMS as a Culture-bound Syndrome', in *Lectures on the Psychology of Women*, ed. by Joan C. Chrisler, Carla Golden, and Patricia D. Rozee (New York: McGraw-Hill, 1996), 106–21, cited in Joan C. Chrisler and Paula Caplan, 'The Strange Case of Dr. Jekyll and Ms. Hyde: How PMS Became a Cultural Phenomenon and a Psychiatric Disorder', *Annual Review of Sex Research*, 13:1 (2002), 274–306 https://doi.org/10.1080/10532528.2002.10559807

252. Chrisler and Caplan, 'The Strange Case of Dr. Jekyll and Ms. Hyde', pp. 276, 292.
253. Shelley Day, 'Puerperal Insanity: The Historical Sociology of a Disease' (unpublished doctoral thesis, Cambridge University, 1985), cited in Natasha Mauthner, 'Towards a Feminist Understanding of Postnatal Depression', *Feminism and Psychology*, 3.3 (1993), 350–55 https://doi.org/10.1177/0959353593033006 p. 351.
254. Mauthner, 'Towards a Feminist Understanding', p. 351.
255. Chloë Taylor, 'Female Sexual Dysfunction, Feminist Sexology, and the Psychiatry of the Normal', *Feminist Studies*, 41.2 (2015), 259–92 https://doi.org/10.15767/feministstudies.41.2.259 p. 286.
256. Susan Bordo, *Unbearable Weight: Feminism, Western Culture, and the Body* (Berkeley: University of California Press, 1993).
Cressida Heyes, 'Diagnosing Culture: Body Dysmorphic Disorder and Cosmetic Surgery', *Body and Society*, 15.4 (2009), 73–93 https://doi.org/10.1177/1357034X09347222
All cited in Taylor, 'Female Sexual Dysfunction', p. 286.
257. Susie Orbach, *Hunger Strike: Starving amidst Plenty* (London and New York: Karnac, 2005), p. 78.
258. Lynne Lamberg, 'Social Phobia—Not Just another Name for Shyness', *Journal of the American Medical Association*, 280.8 (1998), 685–86 https://doi.org/10.1001/jama.280.8.685-JMN0826-3-1
Claudia Kalb, 'Challenging "Extreme" Shyness', *Newsweek* (2003) https://www.newsweek.com/challenging-extreme-shyness-139679 [accessed 7 January 2021].
259. Franklin R. Schneier, Carlos Blanco, Smita X. Antia, and Michael R. Liebowitz, 'The Social Anxiety Spectrum', *Psychiatric Clinics of North America*, 25.4 (2002), 757–74 https://doi.org/10.1016/s0193-953x(02)00018-7

260. John H. Greist, James W. Jefferson, and David Katzelnick, *Social Anxiety Disorder: A Guide* (Madison: Information Centers, Madison Institute of Medicine, 2000), p. 7.
261. Kramer, *Listening to Prozac*, p. 170.
262. Taylor, 'Female Sexual Dysfunction', p. 286.
263. Ussher, 'Diagnosing Difficult Women', p. 66.
264. Mary Ann Jimenez, 'Gender and Psychiatry: Psychiatric Conceptions of Mental Disorders in Women, 1960–1994', *Affilia*, 12.2 (1997), 154–75 https://doi.org/10.1177/088610999701200202
265. Jimenez, 'Gender and Psychiatry', p. 158.
266. Ussher, 'Diagnosing Difficult Women', p. 65.
267. APA, *Diagnostic and Statistical Manual of Mental Disorders*, 3rd edn [*DSM-III*] (Washington DC: American Psychiatric Association Publishing, 1980), p. 348, cited in Ussher, 'Diagnosing Difficult Women', p. 65.
268. Jane M. Ussher, *Fantasies of Femininity: Reframing the Boundaries of Sex* (London/New York: Penguin/Rutgers, 1997), cited in Ussher, 'Diagnosing Difficult Women', p. 65.
269. Erving Goffman, *The Presentation of Self in Everyday Life* (New York: Anchor, 1959), cited in Kathryn A. Ziegler, *'Formidable-Femininity': Performing Gender and Third Wave Feminism in a Women's Self-Defense Class* (Saarbrücken: LAP LAMBERT Academic Publishing, 2010), p. 10.
270. APA, *DSM-5*, p. 429.
271. Ibid., p. 433.
272. Ibid., p. 437.
273. The same study by Laumann and colleagues which I cited earlier on in the chapter.
274. Laumann et al., 'Sexual Dysfunction in the United States', cited in Taylor, 'Female Sexual Dysfunction', pp. 261–62.
275. Taylor, 'Female Sexual Dysfunction', p. 282.
276. Ibid., p. 265.
277. Ibid., p. 285.
278. Ibid., p. 282.
279. Ibid., pp. 283–84.
280. APA, *DSM-5*, p. 202.
281. Anke W. Blöte, Marcia J. W. Kint, Anne C. Miers, and P. Michiel Westenberg, 'The Relation between Public Speaking Anxiety and Social Anxiety: A Review', *Journal of Anxiety Disorders*, 23.3 (2009), 305–13 https://doi.org/10.1016/j.janxdis.2008.11.007
282. APA, *DSM-5*, p. 203.

283. Alec C. Pollard and Gibson J. Henderson, 'Four Types of Social Phobia in a Community Sample', *Journal of Nervous and Mental Disease*, 176.7 (1988), 440–45 https://doi.org/10.1097/00005053-198807000-00006
284. Murray B. Stein, John R. Walker, and David R. Forde, 'Public-speaking Fears in a Community Sample: Prevalence, Impact on Functioning, and Diagnostic Classification', *Archives of General Psychiatry*, 53.2 (1996), 169–74 https://doi.org/10.1001/archpsyc.1996.01830020087010
285. Murray B. Stein, John R. Walker, and David R. Forde, 'Setting Diagnostic Thresholds for Social Phobia', *American Journal of Psychiatry*, 151.3 (1994), 408–12 https://doi.org/10.1176/ajp.151.3.408
286. Philip G. Zimbardo, *Shyness: What It Is, what To Do about It* (Reading, MA: Addison-Wesley, 1977).
287. David J. De Wit, Michelle Chandler-Coutts, David R. Offord, Gillian King, Janette McDougall, Jacqueline Specht, and Shannon Stewart, 'Gender Differences in the Effects of Family Adversity on the Risk of Onset of DSM-III-R Social Phobia', *Journal of Anxiety Disorders*, 19.5 (2005), 479–502 https://doi.org/10.1016/j.janxdis.2004.04.010
    Hans-Ulrich Wittchen, Murray B. Stein, and Ronald C. Kessler, 'Social Fears and Social Phobia in a Community Sample of Adolescents and Young Adults: Prevalence, Risk Factors and Co-morbidity', *Psychological Medicine*, 29.2 (1999), 309–23 https://doi.org/10.1017/s0033291798008174
    Maya Asher, Anu Asnaani, and Idan M. Aderka, 'Gender Differences in Social Anxiety Disorder: A Review', *Clinical Psychology Review*, 56 (2017), 1–12 https://doi.org/10.1016/j.cpr.2017.05.004
288. Kramer, *Listening to Prozac*, p. 270.
289. Ibid., p. 271.
290. Paula J. Caplan, 'Pathologizing your Period', *Ms. Magazine*, 18.3 (2008), 63–64, p. 64.
291. Rome, 'Premenstrual Syndrome (PMS) Examined through a Feminist Lens', p. 145.
292. Browne, 'Is Premenstrual Dysphoric Disorder Really a Disorder?', p. 320.
293. Ibid.
294. Arthur W. Frank, *At the Will of the Body: Reflections on Illness* (Boston: Houghton Mifflin, 1991).
    Rita Schreiber, '(Re)defining my Self: Women's Process of Recovery from Depression', *Qualitative Health Research*, 6.4 (1996), 469–91 https://doi.org/10.1177/104973239600600402
    Damien Ridge and Sue Ziebland, '"The Old Me Could never Have Done that": How People Give Meaning to Recovery Following Depression', *Qualitative Health Research*, 16.8 (2006), 1038–53 https://doi.org/10.1177/1049732306292132

All cited in Browne, 'Is Premenstrual Dysphoric Disorder Really a Disorder?', p. 320.

295. Ibid.
296. Richard G. Tedeschi, Crystal L. Park, and Lawrence G. Calhoun, *Posttraumatic Growth: Positive Changes in the Aftermath of Crisis* (Mahwah, NJ: Lawrence Erlbaum Associates, 1998), cited in Browne, 'Is Premenstrual Dysphoric Disorder Really a Disorder?', p. 320.
297. Erica Leibrandt, *The Surprising Benefits of Having Social Anxiety* https://www.elephantjournal.com/2016/05/the-surprising-benefits-of-having-social-anxiety/ [accessed 6 September 2019].
298. Royal College of Psychiatrists, *Shyness and Social Phobia* (2016) https://www.rcpsych.ac.uk/mental-health/problems-disorders/shyness-and-social-phobia [accessed 6 September 2019].
299. M. Altmann, E. Knowles, and H. Bull, 'A Psychosomatic Study of the Sex Cycle in Women', *Psychosomatic Medicine*, 3.3 (1941), 199–225 https://doi.org/10.1097/00006842-194107000-00001

    Melville E. Ivey, M. E. and Judith M. Bardwick, 'Patterns of Affective Fluctuation in the Menstrual Cycle', *Psychosomatic Medicine*, 30.3 (1968), 336–45 https://doi.org/10.1097/00006842-196805000-00008

    All cited in Jacquelyn N. Zita, 'The Premenstrual Syndrome: "Dis-easing" the Female Cycle', *Hypatia*, 3.1 (1988), 77–99 https://doi.org/10.1111/j.1527-2001.1988.tb00057.x
300. Chrisler and Caplan, 'The Strange Case of Dr. Jekyll and Ms. Hyde', p. 276.
301. Jane M. Ussher, 'The Role of Premenstrual Dysphoric Disorder in the Subjectification of Women', *Journal of Medical Humanities*, 24 (2003), 131–46 https://doi.org/10.1023/A:1021366001305 p. 136.
302. Chrisler, 'PMS as a Culture-bound Syndrome', cited in Chrisler and Caplan, 'The Strange Case of Dr. Jekyll and Ms. Hyde', p. 279.
303. Laumann et al., 'Sexual Dysfunction in the United States', cited in Judy Z. Segal, 'The Rhetoric of Female Sexual Dysfunction: Faux Feminism and the FDA', *Canadian Medical Association Journal*, 187.12 (2015), 915–16 https://doi.org/10.1503/cmaj.150363 p. 916.
304. Sprout Pharmaceuticals, *Home Page* (2019) www.sproutpharma.com [accessed 29 June 2015], cited in Segal, 'The Rhetoric of Female Sexual Dysfunction', p. 916.
305. Mara Schiavocampo, Jackie Jesko, and Lauren Effron, 'Fight over "Little Pink Pill" Raises Sexism Questions', *ABC News* (2014) https://abcnews.go.com/Health/fight-pink-pill-boosting-womens-sex-drive-raises/story?id=23813586 [accessed 7 January 2021].

    All cited in Segal, 'The Rhetoric of Female Sexual Dysfunction', p. 916.
306. Segal, 'The Rhetoric of Female Sexual Dysfunction', p. 916.

307. Ibid.
308. Ibid.
309. Lisa Cosgrove, 'Crying out Loud: Understanding Women's Emotional Distress as both Lived Experience and Social Construction', *Feminism and Psychology*, 10.2 (2000), 247–67 https://doi.org/10.1177/0959353500010002004 cited in Jane M. Ussher and Janette Perz, 'PMS as a Gendered Illness Linked to the Construction and Relational Experience of Hetero-femininity', *Sex Roles*, 68.1–2 (2013), 132–50 https://doi.org/10.1007/s11199-011-9977-5 p. 133.
310. Chrisler and Caplan, 'The Strange Case of Dr. Jekyll and Ms. Hyde', cited in Ussher, 'Diagnosing Difficult Women', p. 67.
311. Anne E. Figert, 'Premenstrual Syndrome as Scientific and Cultural Artifact', *Integrative Physiological and Behavioral Science*, 40.2 (2005), 102–13 https://doi.org/10.1007/BF02734245 p. 67.
312. Mary B. Parlee, 'The Premenstrual Syndrome', *Psychological Bulletin*, 80.6 (1973), 454–65 https://doi.org/10.1037/h0035270 cited in Ussher, 'Diagnosing Difficult Women', p. 67.
313. Ussher, 'The Role of Premenstrual Dysphoric Disorder', pp. 132–33.
314. Susan H. McDaniel, 'The Interpersonal Politics of Premenstrual Syndrome', *Family Systems Medicine*, 6.2 (1988), 134–49 https://doi.org/10.1037/h0089741

     Chrisler and Caplan, 'The Strange Case of Dr. Jekyll and Ms. Hyde', pp. 276, 288.
315. Figert, 'Premenstrual Syndrome as Scientific and Cultural Artifact', pp. 104–05.

     Anne L. Stout and John F. Steege, 'Psychological Assessment of Women Seeking Treatment for Premenstrual Syndrome', *Journal of Psychosomatic Research*, 29.6 (1985), 621–29 https://doi.org/10.1016/0022-3999(85)90071-6 cited in Ussher and Perz, 'PMS as a Gendered Illness', p. 135.
316. Johnson and Kandrack, 'On the Medico-legal Appropriation of Menstrual Discourse', p. 25.
317. Diane N. Ruble and Jeanne Brooks-Gunn, 'Menstrual Symptoms: A Social Cognition Analysis', *Journal of Behavioral Medicine*, 2.2 (1979), 171–94 https://doi.org/10.1007/BF00846665 cited in Loes Knaapen and George Weisz, 'The Biomedical Standardization of Premenstrual Syndrome', *Studies in History and Philosophy of Science. Part C: Studies in History and Philosophy of Biological and Biomedical Sciences*, 39.1 (2008), 120–34 https://doi.org/10.1016/j.shpsc.2007.12.009 p. 126.
318. Johnson and Kandrack, 'On the Medico-legal Appropriation of Menstrual Discourse', pp. 25, 26.
319. Chrisler and Caplan, 'The Strange Case of Dr. Jekyll and Ms. Hyde', pp. 276, 288.

Marion Pirie, 'Women and the Illness Role: Rethinking Feminist Theory', *Canadian Review of Sociology and Anthropology*, 25.4 (1988), 628–48 https://doi.org/10.1111/j.1755-618X.1988.tb00123.x p. 642, cited in Browne, 'Is Premenstrual Dysphoric Disorder Really a Disorder?', p. 320.
McDaniel, 'The Interpersonal Politics of Premenstrual Syndrome', cited in Ussher and Perz, 'PMS as a Gendered Illness', p. 135.

320. Caplan, 'Pathologizing your Period', p. 64.
321. Ussher, 'The Role of Premenstrual Dysphoric Disorder', cited in Ussher and Perz, 'PMS as a Gendered Illness', p. 140.
322. Ibid.
323. Joan C. Chrisler, 'How To Regain your Control and Balance: The "Pop" Approach to PMS', Manuscript under review (2001), cited in Chrisler and Caplan, 'The Strange Case of Dr. Jekyll and Ms. Hyde', p. 276, 288.
324. Cosgrove, 'Crying out Loud'.
    Janet Lee and Jennifer Sasser-Coen, *Blood Stories: Menarche and the Politics of the Female Body in Contemporary US Society* (New York: Routledge, 1996).
    Jane M. Ussher, 'Premenstrual Syndrome and Self-policing: Ruptures in Self-silencing Leading to Increased Self-surveillance and Blaming of the Body', *Social Theory and Health*, 2 (2004), 254–72 https://doi.org/10.1057/palgrave.sth.8700032
    Jane M. Ussher, Myra S. Hunter, and S. J. Browne, 'Good, Bad or Dangerous To Know: Representations of Femininity in Narrative Accounts of PMS', in *Culture and Psychology*, ed. by Corinne Squire (Falmer: Routledge, 2000), 87–99.
    All cited in Ussher and Perz, 'PMS as a Gendered Illness', p. 136.
325. Sophie Laws, 'The Sexual Politics of Premenstrual Tension', *Women's Studies International Forum*, 6.1 (1983), 19–31 https://doi.org/10.1016/0277-5395(83)90084-5 cited in Chrisler and Caplan, 'The Strange Case of Dr. Jekyll and Ms. Hyde', p. 289.
326. L. Cosgrove and B. Riddle, 'Constructions of Femininity and Experiences of Menstrual Distress', *Women and Health* (in press), cited in Chrisler and Caplan, 'The Strange Case of Dr. Jekyll and Ms. Hyde', p. 289.
327. K. Berggren-Clive, 'Out of the Darkness and into the Light: Women's Experiences with Depression after Childbirth', *Canadian Journal of Community Mental Health*, 17.1 (1998), 103–20 https://doi.org/10.7870/cjcmh-1998-0006
    Natasha Mauthner, '"I Wasn't Being True to Myself". Women's Narratives of Postpartum Depression', in *The Depression Epidemic: International Perspectives on Women's Self-silencing and Psychological Distress*, ed. by Dana Crowley Jack and Alisha Ali (Oxford: Oxford University Press, 2010), 459–84.
    All cited in Ussher and Perz, 'PMS as a Gendered Illness', p. 137.

328. Mauthner, '"I Wasn't Being True to Myself", p. 470, cited in Ussher and Perz, 'PMS as a Gendered Illness', p. 137.
329. Mark Epstein, *Thoughts without a Thinker: Psychotherapy from a Buddhist Perspective* (London: Duckworth, 1996), p. 144, cited in Ussher, 'The Role of Premenstrual Dysphoric Disorder', pp. 137–38.
330. Ussher, 'The Role of Premenstrual Dysphoric Disorder', pp. 137–38.
331. Katie Masters, 'An Analysis of Women and Social Anxiety Disorder from the Perspectives of Feminism and Anti-psychiatry' (unpublished Master of Research thesis, University of Birmingham, 2016).
332. Michel Foucault, *History of Madness*, p. 25.
333. Michel Foucault, *Discipline and Punish [Surveiller et Punir]* trans. Alan Sheridan (Harmondsworth: Penguin, 1991[1975]).
334. Foucault, *Discipline and Punish*, p. 200.
335. Ibid., p. 202.
336. Michel Foucault, *Power/Knowledge: Selected Interviews and other Writings, 1972–1977*, ed. by Colin Gordon, (New York: Pantheon Books, 1980), p. 131.
337. Ussher and Perz, 'PMS as a Gendered Illness', p. 138.
338. Ussher, 'Premenstrual Syndrome and Self-policing'.
Ussher and Perz, 'PMS as a Gendered Illness', p. 138.
339. Dana Crowley Jack, *Silencing the Self: Women and Depression* (Cambridge, MA: Harvard University Press, 1991).
Helen O'Grady, *Woman's Relationship with Herself: Gender, Foucault, Therapy* (London: Routledge, 2005).
All cited in Ussher and Perz, 'PMS as a Gendered Illness', p. 136.
340. Paula J. Caplan, *The Myth of Women's Masochism* (Lincoln, Nebraska: iUniverse, 2005), p. 11.
341. Jean Grimshaw, *Philosophy and Feminist Thinking* (Minneapolis: University of Minnesota Press, 1986), p. 196.
342. Ussher and Perz, 'PMS as a Gendered Illness', p. 136.
343. Ibid.
344. Janette Perz and Jane M. Ussher, 'Women's Experience of Premenstrual Change: A Case of Silencing the Self', *Journal of Reproductive and Infant Psychology*, 24.4 (2006), 289–303 https://doi.org/10.1080/02646830600973883
Ussher, 'Premenstrual Syndrome and Self-policing'.
Jane M. Ussher and Janette Perz, 'Disruption of the Silenced-self: The Case of Pre-menstrual Syndrome', in Jack and Ali, *The Depression Epidemic*, 435–58.
345. Jack, *Silencing the Self: Women and Depression.*
346. Dana Crowley Jack, 'The Silencing the Self Scale', *Fairhaven Faculty Publications* (2017), 14 https://cedar.wwu.edu/cgi/viewcontent.cgi?article=1013&context=fairhaven_facpubs [accessed 24 April 2023].

347. Dana Crowley Jack and Diana Dill, 'The Silencing the Self Scale: Schemas of Intimacy with Depression in Women', *Psychology of Women Quarterly*, 16.1 (1992), 97–106 https://doi.org/10.1111/j.1471-6402.1992.tb00242.x p. 98.
Ussher and Perz, 'PMS as a Gendered Illness', p. 135.
348. Jack and Dill, 'The Silencing the Self Scale', p. 98.
Ussher and Perz, 'PMS as a Gendered Illness', p. 135.
349. Laing, *The Divided Self.*
350. Masters, 'An Analysis of Women and Social Anxiety Disorder'.
351. Laing, quoted in Chang, *Wisdom for the Soul*, p. 412.
352. Janet Stoppard, *Understanding Depression: Feminist Social Constructionist Approaches* (London: Routledge, 2014), cited in Browne, 'Is Premenstrual Dysphoric Disorder Really a Disorder?', p. 323.
353. Ussher and Perz, 'PMS as a Gendered Illness', p. 140.
354. Chrisler and Johnston-Robledo, 'Raging Hormones?', cited in Chrisler and Caplan, 'The Strange Case of Dr. Jekyll and Ms. Hyde', pp. 276, 277.
355. Alisha Ali, Paula J. Caplan, and Rachel Fagnant, 'Gender Stereotypes in Diagnostic Criteria', in *Handbook of Gender Research in Psychology, Vol. 2: Gender Research in Social and Applied Psychology*, ed. by Joan C. Chrisler and Donald R. McCreary (New York: Springer, 2010), 91–109, cited in Browne, 'Is Premenstrual Dysphoric Disorder Really a Disorder?', p. 322.
356. Jane M. Ussher, *The Madness of Women: Myth and Experience* (London: Routledge, 2011).
357. Ussher, 'Diagnosing Difficult Women', p. 66.
358. McInnes, 'The Political Is Personal'.
359. Zita, 'The Premenstrual Syndrome', p. 90.
360. Chrisler and Caplan, 'The Strange Case of Dr. Jekyll and Ms. Hyde', pp. 276, 296.
361. British Psychological Society, *Response to the American Psychiatric Association: DSM-5 Development* (2011) http://apps.bps.org.uk/_publicationfiles/consultation-responses/DSM-5%202011%20-%20BPS%20response.pdf cited in Browne, 'Is Premenstrual Dysphoric Disorder Really a Disorder?', p. 317.
362. Jane M. Ussher, *The Psychology of the Female Body* (London: Routledge, 1989), p. 73, cited in Figert, 'Premenstrual Syndrome as Scientific and Cultural Artifact', pp. 104–05.
363. Chrisler and Caplan, 'The Strange Case of Dr. Jekyll and Ms. Hyde', p. 283.
364. Susan Gair, 'Distress and Depression in New Motherhood: Research with Adoptive Mothers Highlights Important Contributing Factors', *Child and Family Social Work*, 4.1 (1999) https://doi.org/10.1046/j.1365-2206.1999.00098.x p. 56.
365. Karen B. Levy, *The Politics of Women's Health Care: Medicalization as a Form of Social Control* (Mesquite, TX: Ide House, 1993).

Catherine K. Riessman, 'Women and Medicalization: A New Perspective', *Social Policy*, 14.1 (1983), 3–18 https://pubmed.ncbi.nlm.nih.gov/10264493/ [accessed 5 January 2021].
Susan S. M. Edwards, *Women on Trial: A Study of the Female Suspect, Defendant and Offender in the Criminal Law and Criminal Justice System* (Dover: Manchester University Press, 1984).
Sophie Laws, Valerie Hey, and Andrea Egan, *Seeing Red: The Politics of Pre-menstrual Tension* (London: Hutchinson, 1985).

366. Laws, *Issues of Blood*, cited in Ussher, 'Premenstrual Syndrome: Reconciling Disciplinary Divides', pp. 225, 235.
367. Browne, 'Is Premenstrual Dysphoric Disorder Really a Disorder?', p. 318.
368. Mauthner, 'Towards a Feminist Understanding', p. 352.
369. Kathy Kendall, 'The Politics of Premenstrual Syndrome: Implications for Feminist Justice', *The Journal of Human Justice*, 2.2 (1991), 77–98 https://doi.org/10.1007/BF02636788 p. 91, cited in Johnson and Kandrack, 'On the Medico-legal Appropriation of Menstrual Discourse', p. 25.
370. Mauthner, 'Towards a Feminist Understanding', p. 352.
371. Ussher, 'Premenstrual Syndrome: Reconciling Disciplinary Divides', p. 226.
372. Chrisler and Caplan, 'The Strange Case of Dr. Jekyll and Ms. Hyde', p. 298.
373. Browne, 'Is Premenstrual Dysphoric Disorder Really a Disorder?', p. 316.
374. Ibid.
375. Riessman, 'Women and Medicalization'.
Edwards, *Women on Trial.*
Laws et al., *Seeing Red*, cited in Browne, 'Is Premenstrual Dysphoric Disorder Really a Disorder?', p. 320.
376. Browne, 'Is Premenstrual Dysphoric Disorder Really a Disorder?', p. 317.
377. Qing Li, Xiaoming Li, and Bonita Stanton, 'Alcohol Use among Female Sex Workers and Male Clients: An Integrative Review of Global Literature', *Alcohol and Alcoholism*, 45.2 (2010), 188–99 https://doi.org/10.1093/alcalc/agp095 cited in Browne, 'Is Premenstrual Dysphoric Disorder Really a Disorder?', p. 318.
378. Ellyn Kaschak and Leonore Tiefer (eds.), *A New View of Women's Sexual Problems* (New York: Haworth Press, 2001).
Also see Leonore Tiefer, *The New View Manifesto* (2000) http://www.newviewcampaign.org/manifesto.asp [accessed 26 September 2020].
379. Tiefer, *The New View Manifesto.*
380. Ibid.
381. Katherine Angel, 'Contested Psychiatric Ontology and Feminist Critique: "Female Sexual Dysfunction" and the Diagnostic and Statistical Manual', *History of the Human Sciences*, 25.4 (2012), 3–24 https://doi.org/10.1177/0952695112456949 p. 12.

382. Boston Women's Health Collective, 'How Real Is PMS?', *Ms.*, III.4 (1992), 75–76, cited in Figert, 'Premenstrual Syndrome as Scientific and Cultural Artifact', p. 107.
383. Ussher, 'Premenstrual Syndrome: Reconciling Disciplinary Divides', p. 238.
384. Elizabeth Mollard, 'Exploring Paradigms in Postpartum Depression Research: The Need for Feminist Pragmatism', *Health Care for Women International*, 36.4 (2015), 378–91 https://doi.org/10.1080/07399332.2014.903951 pp. 382, 378–91, 382–83, 385, 386.
385. Ussher, 'Premenstrual Syndrome: Reconciling Disciplinary Divides', p. 244.
386. Mollard, 'Exploring Paradigms in Postpartum Depression Research', pp. 383, 388.
387. Ibid., p. 388.
388. WHO, 'Social Phobias'.
389. Royal College of Psychiatrists, 'Shyness and Social Phobia'.

CHAPTER 3

'Co-morbidities', Femininities, and Non-normativities

This chapter opens by exploring participants' experiences of both seeking and not seeking help for their mental distress. In many cases, their mental distress was not restricted to social anxiety, but bled into other forms—'co-morbidities', in psychiatric terms—such as eating problems and sadness. Placing this aspect of interviewees' narratives into dialogue with the *DSM-5*'s account of the interplay between SAD and other diagnoses has two effects. Firstly, it highlights the poor demarcation between diagnostic categories, thereby problematising the purported objective nature of them as disease entities. Secondly, it raises the possibility that non-normativity—routes to which include neurodiversity, personality style, and physical health conditions—gives rise to experiencing social anxiety. As such, 'co-morbidities' form a backdrop not only to this entire chapter, but to the entire book. Discussing the role of physical health conditions then provides a springboard from which to dive into the chapter's final portion, wherein I home in on physicality. That is, examining participants' encounters with microaggressions and their effects on the body offers a means by which we can explore how mental distress is experienced by the woman in her entirety. In turn, through utilising feminist scholarship on embodiment, a holistic understanding of women's social anxiety is presented.

K. Masters, *Feminist and Anti-Psychiatry Perspectives on 'Social Anxiety Disorder'*,
https://doi.org/10.1007/978-3-031-48707-1_3

(Not) Seeking Help and 'Co-morbidities'

All of the women I interviewed had sought medical help for their mental distress, although none of them had sought help for social anxiety in isolation. Indeed, only Olivia and Farah had even mentioned their social anxiety to their doctors. Accordingly, other types of mental distress had formed the basis of help-seeking for everybody else. For Ria and Daniella, this was for eating problems; for Phoebe, it was for nervousness. For Amy, it was for nervousness and sadness; for Ellen, it was for sadness.

Since we are discussing help-seeking, it is worth revisiting Talcott Parsons's 'sick role'. One key requirement of entering this role is 'the obligation […] to seek *technically competent* help, namely […] that of a physician and to *cooperate* with him in […] trying to get well'.[1] A number of the women I interviewed had only sought help when their mental distress was incapacitating or had been endured for a long time—sometimes both. Daniella's narrative on her eating problems exemplified this, since she told me: '[M]y first two and a half years of the PhD were really low […] I couldn't function properly […] I could not get out of bed.' And Phoebe's description of feeling panicked on waking every day communicated overwhelming distress: '[I]t's like crushing on your chest […] like [gasps] "Oh my God! […] I can't breathe."'

On mental distress that is incapacitating, there is a link to be made with Parsons's thoughts on illness, functionality, and society. He proposes that 'health is included in the functional needs of the individual member of the society' and that 'illness incapacitates for the effective performance of social roles'.[2] Perhaps participants sought help only when their mental distress became incapacitating because this was the point at which it affected their functionality and resulting fulfilling of their social roles. This is convincing in the case of socially anxious women in particular if we consider sociologist Matthias Zick Varul's contention that '[f]ailure to fulfil role expectations […] incurs the risk of social exclusion'.[3]

My impression that some participants had been reluctant to seek help was borne out when they told me that, when they eventually did so, it was only because they had been persuaded to by others. Ellen told me: '[I]t's only because my dad dragged me to the doctors.' Likewise, Olivia said: '[I]t was my boyfriend who encouraged me to seek help.' As Parsons observes, it is often others who define that the patient is sick[4] and, in turn, grant access to the sick role.[5] For *women*, that their help-seeking seems to be at the behest of others evokes feminist psychotherapists Susie Orbach and Luise Eichenbaum's thoughts on women in our society: '[S]he must *defer* to others, follow their lead, articulate her needs only in relation to theirs.'[6]

Having contemplated why women might be hesitant vis-à-vis help-seeking for mental distress in general, there might be further reasons in considering social anxiety specifically. For me, the nature of social anxiety itself presents difficulties at every step: having to psych myself up to make the telephone call to book the appointment; sitting in a busy waiting room where I feel like all eyes are on me; and then disclosing personal and upsetting experiences to a stranger in a clinical setting, all the while conscious of not overshooting my allotted time. But what arose when I began interviewing the women was something else: some of them refuted social anxiety's characterisation as a disorder.[7] Ellen remarked: 'I've never said I have "Social Anxiety Disorder", I've just said I would [be] anxious with certain things.' Farah's narrative went a step further in that it spoke to the idea that social anxiety should be viewed as just another element of one's personality:[8]

> Why should I [...] [b]e calm, all the time[?] [...] Maybe it's not a bad thing if I have this experience [...] we can really embrace different images in society [...] and we don't need [...] to have just one good image of a successful person.

Ellen's and Farah's accounts bespeak a resistance to entering the sick role: in rejecting the conceptualisation of their social anxiety as illness, they are disobeying the requirement that they should 'want to "get well"'.[9] Parsons proposes that illness is already 'a type of deviant behavior'[10] insofar as the sick individual is one who 'avoid[s] conforming with the normative standards of the common culture [...] and he resists social pressures to bring him back "in line"'.[11] By eschewing the sick role, the already-deviant socially anxious woman is then *doubly* deviant, for, as author and academic Molly McKinney articulates, she is viewed as an incompliant patient determined towards the destruction of both herself and society.[12]

Having established that there might be reluctance among socially anxious women to seek help, and that help is usually sought for other forms of mental distress, the interplay between social anxiety and these other forms warrants further examination. The *DSM-5* states that 'the onset of social anxiety disorder generally precedes that of the other disorders'.[13] Put another way, social anxiety comes first, the implication being that it might *cause* other forms of mental distress. But is the reverse possible? Could it be that a nervous or subdued temperament exposes a woman to the social conditions which contribute to worries about others' judgements? Indeed, exhibiting *any* characteristic which society views as non-normative could promote this since, as disability scholar Lennard J. Davis notes, 'The concept of a norm [...] implies that the majority of the population must or should somehow be part of the norm.'[14] As such, divergence from normativity can bring about interactions with others which are conducive to experiencing mental distress. These might comprise ridicule and humiliation, being paid undue attention, feeling as though one is being watched, and having a sense of not belonging or being an outsider. Protagonist Meursault in Albert Camus's *L'Étranger* sums up these feelings rather well when he says: 'I felt the urge to reassure him that I was like everybody else, just like everybody else.'[15]

Davis's remark on conforming to the norm has elements in common with the writing of psychiatric survivor activist Judi Chamberlin. Chamberlin notes that 'the public dislikes mental patients, mentally retarded people, the physically disabled, the deformed or disfigured'.[16] To borrow Camus's phrasing, the public dislikes those who are decidedly *not* like everybody else. Applying this to mental distress, Chamberlin coins the term 'mentalism', that is, 'the unreasonable fear of mental patients'.[17] While Chamberlin deploys this concept in writing about those who have been detained as inpatients, her concept also has utility in considering the experiences of socially anxious women.[18] Chamberlin puts forth that '[n]egative stereotypes of the "mentally ill" are everywhere and are difficult not to internalize, no matter how sensitive one becomes'.[19] One of the buttresses of mentalism is that it is 'built into the language—*sick* and *crazy* are widely used to refer to behavior of which the speaker disapproves'.[20] Crucially, 'Like racism and sexism, mentalism infects its victims with the belief in their own inferiority.'[21]

Merging the thoughts of the anti-psychiatrists[22] with strands from Davis's disability studies and Chamberlin's mentalism, I wonder whether SAD is an intelligible phenomenon arising from how 'an ableist society that places a great premium on being "normal"'[23] treats women who are *non*-normative. Taking inspiration from the social model of disability, we might then conceptualise these women's social anxiety as 'a social creation' as opposed to endorsing the medical conceptualisation of it as an 'individual deficit'.[24]

Following on from this, I want to move my attention to Phoebe. Near to the beginning of our interview, Phoebe told me that she strongly suspects that she is autistic. This took me aback, since, although I had not (yet) mentioned this to Phoebe, in the few months prior to our interview I had had the same inkling about myself. The diagnosis 'Autism Spectrum Disorder' (ASD) is distinct from what are classified as 'Psychiatric Disorders'—Anxiety, Depression, SAD—in that it is characterised as a 'Neurodevelopmental Disorder': it is said to affect the brain and central nervous system.[25] With that said, scholars Erika Dyck and Ginny Russell raise important points in telling us that

> Autism is not currently identified by neurological markers as none are reliable enough to create diagnostic tests [...] it is behavioural inventories that are used to diagnose ASD, not brain scans, and these use a dimensional scale of impairment with a cut-off rather than a dichotomous distinction. In the diagnostic process, the point at which individual differences in behaviour constitute autism is based on clinical decisions which may depend on resources that diagnosis will trigger, the meaning of diagnosis to the patient[,] or clinicians' own ideas about signs and signifiers of autism. Thus, a somewhat arbitrary cut-off is used on the autism spectrum to define autism as a diagnosed disorder. This process is heavily influenced by culture, context, and values.[26]

Therefore, despite its categorisation as a Neurodevelopmental Disorder, ASD is subject to the same critique as psychiatric diagnoses. That is, while the *DSM-5*'s conceptualisation of ASD holds that it arises from biological malfunction in the brain and nervous system, its diagnosis hinges on cultural norms. It is perhaps then rather fitting that Neurodevelopmental Disorders come under the remit of psychiatry: they feature in the *DSM-5*[27] and *ICD-10*,[28] and diagnosis and management of ASD in the UK will involve a psychiatrist.[29]

As opposed to subscribing to the *DSM-5*'s conception of ASD—as a disease entity or 'a deficit-based description of a person'[30]—I instead look to the neurodiversity movement's conception of this diagnosis. This echoes tenets from disability studies, such as Davis's writings on 'the variability of the body',[31] with the population comprising 'a continuum of physical differences'.[32] Analogously, I posit that ASD should be considered 'in terms of the normal variation of the human population'[33] and as a valid 'way of being'.[34]

Returning to the *DSM-5*'s commentary on ASD, the manual tells us that 'about 70% of individuals with autism spectrum disorder may have one comorbid mental disorder, and 40% may have two or more comorbid mental disorders',[35] examples of which include Anxiety Disorders.[36] Phoebe speaks to this intertwinement in saying, 'I think all my anxiety stems from like relationships with other people […] I actually think […] I'm autistic.' Relationships with other people are at the root of Phoebe's anxieties, but she seems not to attribute this to her SAD, but to her autism. This calls into question the idea that social anxiety precedes—and the possibility that it therefore triggers—the development of 'co-morbid' psychiatric disorders. Instead, Phoebe's narrative suggests that social anxiety arises from others' reactions to non-normative temperaments or ways of being. On this point, Phoebe told me that being autistic makes her feel like an outsider, for she feels fundamentally different from others: 'I don't feel like my brain is like the same as other people's.'

Although she did not disclose whether or not she is autistic, Amy's testimony evoked how Phoebe spoke about her brain. Specifically, Amy explained how everything is coloured by her mental distress:

> It permeates every part of your life […] My mental illness is inside my friendships and it's in my home and it's in my work, but—no, it's not in any of those, it's inside my brain and it just feels like it's everywhere because I have to filter my experience of life through my brain.

Amy's and Phoebe's narratives indicate that their dispositions and lived experiences of mental distress shape their outlooks. Indeed, as psychologist Derald Wing Sue notes, 'How one views the world […] serves as a prism from which data and information are filtered.'[37] Experiencing the world differently from others, no matter to what this is attributable, may foster social anxiety by creating a sense of estrangement. Phoebe elaborated on how this had played out for her in the past in telling me, '"Oh, I was anxious as a kid." But I thought that that was just how everyone felt.'

In assuming that others experience the world in the same way as do we, Phoebe's words bring to mind author and psychoanalyst Marion Milner's exposition of experiments in childhood development:

> [A] child is not born knowing that what goes on in his own mind has not the same sort of independent existence as what goes on around him. He does not know that a feeling in his own mind is only his feeling, he has no

means of telling, for instance, that the whole world is not darkened with his misery.[38]

Milner goes on to tell us that '[a] child gradually discovers [...] that what is in his mind is not necessarily in other people's'.[39] I cannot help but wonder whether, at least for non-normative women like Phoebe, this discovery remains unexposed for longer than is typical. Perhaps women like Phoebe go on believing that others think in the same way as do they and then struggle to comprehend why others behave in seemingly incomprehensible ways. Phoebe elaborated on how she used to worry as a child, telling me, 'I just remember [...] thinking that that's what everyone did, but then you realise, "Look... It's not."' Realisations such as these might well promote alienation and perhaps, down the road, concern about others' perceptions.

As Phoebe's remarks about her childhood allude to relating to others—or rather, *not* relating to others—both her and Ria spoke further in this area, their anecdotes about interacting with others invoking Sue's construct 'microaggressions'. Consistently experienced by those who are minoritised, microaggressions are defined as 'the constant and continuing everyday reality of slights, insults, invalidations, and indignities visited upon marginalized groups by well-intentioned, moral, and decent family members, friends, neighbours, co-workers, students, teachers, clerks, waiters and waitresses, employers, health care professionals, and educators'.[40] Sue explains that the harm from microaggressions is often psychological, is implicated 'in restricting career and job choices, in creating a lower standard of living [...] and in perpetuating inequities in employment and health care'.[41]

Most pertinent to this book, there is a subset of microaggressions called *gender* microaggressions. These are 'brief and commonplace daily verbal or behavioral indignities, whether intentional or unintentional, that communicate hostile, derogatory, or negative gender slights and insults that potentially have a harmful impact on women'.[42] Phoebe's and Ria's testimonies both featured examples of gender microaggressions which are germane to social anxiety in that they centre on others' opinions of them, and how these are voiced:

Ria: [I]f you went round to someone's house and you were really agreeable and helpful [...] you'd feel as though it would be noted [...] you hear it being talked about [...] I'll chat to my auntie and she'll mention the fact

> that my cousin hasn't sort of got into contact with her in a while [...] that [...] wouldn't even figure for a guy [...] they're cut a bit more slack.

> Phoebe: The fucking boys at our school were such misogynistic little pricks. [...] I remember there was this girl called Lindsey [...] And I remember them [...] making like stomping noises and like shouting at her and then telling her to like, 'Go back to the canteen,' because that's where she should be, kind of thing, because she just wants to eat [...] I remember thinking, 'Oh, if they say that about her, what do they say about me?'

Crucially, Phoebe spoke to the psychological harm of microaggressions in divulging their lasting effect on her:

> And the way they would talk to us, and the other girls, was so disgusting, and you look back and you're like, 'Fuck, no wonder I'm really anxious', because these boys just thought they could talk about girls however they wanted and you just felt like you had to take it [...] you internalise that misogyny and then you carry that with you throughout your life [...] I just think like stuff like that and I'm like, 'No wonder women are so anxious.'

Phoebe's and Ria's experiences of microaggressions seem to have planted a seed in their minds: that they should care about others' impressions of them. In turn, perhaps this has cultivated their social anxiety. Their anecdotes also point to a wider cultural phenomenon: that women are to be openly discussed and evaluated.

When people with marginalised identities experience microaggressions such as these, Sue contends, they use their prior experience 'to add meaning to interpersonal encounters: that is, they evaluate similar experiences they have encountered over time and in different places'.[43] In doing so, individuals often conclude that the linkage between these multiple experiences is the aspect of their identity that renders them minoritised,[44] such as their gender or race. Diverging from Sue's analysis, is it possible that women might attribute the consistency with which they encounter microaggressions not to their gender, or even to the nexus of their interlocking subordinations, but to themselves *as individuals*? This seems probable when microaggressions are not readily linked to an aspect of one's marginalised identity,[45] as might be the case in childhood: girls are not necessarily equipped with the knowledge or critical thinking skills to understand that what happens to them might be the result of structural inequalities, such as institutionalised sexism, as opposed to their individual 'faults'. Daniella's and Farah's stories suggest that they had both experienced microaggressions as children:

> Daniella: I remember going to my first year at school [...] I really didn't get along and I got bullied.
>
> Farah: [M]y sister [...] [was] 13 year[s] [...] older... And my brother [was] 8 years older and all of my cousins were around that age, so I [...] [wasn't] accepted easily in[to] that teenager group [...] I was a sort of outsider.

These narratives feature a recurring theme in interviewees' stories: alienation. It follows that the reverse, belonging, was recurrent in participants' conceptions of social anxiety. For instance, Daniella described changing schools as a teenager, where 'habits were different and kids were different and mentality-wise it was different [...] I always felt out of place'. Similarly, Farah told me that her 'anxiety is related to the feeling of belonging'. She continued:

> I think in my case as an immigrant [...] when you would consider yourself a sort of minority, whether as a woman, or because of your race, ethnicity, [...] sexual orientation or whatever... You would definitely feel that anxiety because you have to struggle to be accepted.

Farah's relating of her experience resonates with the work of psychologists Kay Deaux and Ronni Michelle Greenwood on the intersection of gender and immigration. Most pertinent to Farah's narrative, they write that the immigrant's day-to-day experience comprises 'interactions with the outgroup, where the immigrant confronts and is assessed by members of the host culture'.[46]

Belonging was also a motif in my interview with Ria, who comes from a British-Punjabi family. When we were discussing public speaking, she told me: '[Y]ou might stand up [...] to give a talk—and you get this awareness that maybe you don't belong there.' Writer Gloria Anzaldúa's theorising in her book *Borderlands* is relevant to both Ria's and Farah's mixed ethnicities and multiple identities. In her opus, which draws on the author's lived experience as a Chicano woman, Anzaldúa proposes that

> Living on borders and in margins, keeping intact one's shifting and multiple identity and integrity, is like trying to swim in a new element, an 'alien'

> element [...] the 'alien' element has become familiar—never comfortable, not with society's clamor to uphold the old, to rejoin the flock, to go with the herd.[47]

Participants' rich crosscutting of identities—experiences of mental distress, neurodiversity, immigration status, race, ethnicity—might create for them a sense of not belonging in their containing society. So too might prior experiences: both those that are readily linked to intersecting axes of oppression but *especially* those that are not, such as those described by Daniella and Farah from their childhoods—women might instead ascribe these to their individual 'inadequacies'. Ria succinctly communicated the upshot of all of this in stating that 'the idea that you don't belong [...] can feed social anxiety'.

Phoebe's experiences of autism, on which I touched earlier, are also associated with belonging. '[H]igh-functioning autism' is one of the diagnoses that the *DSM-5* lists as being 'co-morbid' with SAD[48]—I will discuss the other diagnoses in due course. For now, I suggest that the link between social anxiety and autism is more obvious than the link between social anxiety and other 'co-morbidities'. This is because ASD, like social anxiety, is strongly related to interaction. The NHS lists 'seeming blunt, rude or not interested in others without meaning to' and 'not understanding social "rules", such as not talking over people' as common signs of ASD in adults.[49] Since women are, as Phoebe said, 'always told to be like polite and good', a woman exhibiting these signs is not likely to provoke a favourable reaction from others. Phoebe felt the fallout of this in that she would

> [J]ust obsess about my impact on other people to a point where it causes me like quite a lot of turmoil [...] I get so obsessed about things I've said and things I've done, all like, "Oh God, why did I say that?"

In the case of women like Phoebe, we might frame social anxiety as an understandable response to how *others* respond to neurodivergent ways of interacting.

SAD is also cited by the *DSM-5* as being 'co-morbid' with another diagnosis which comprises non-normative interaction: Selective Mutism (SM).[50] As all but one of the participants was interviewed verbally, with Olivia expressing a preference for being interviewed by email, it follows that none of them divulged that they had experienced significant barriers in speaking. The exception to this was Farah, who told of experiencing difficulty communicating in an unfamiliar circumstance:[51] '[I]n the class, I couldn't participate and whenever I wanted to say something, my heartbeat was... In a way that I couldn't breathe, so you can't even talk.' Farah's words evoke one of Anzaldúa's depictions in *Borderlands*:

> Alienated from her mother culture, 'alien' in the dominant culture, the woman of color does not feel safe within the inner life of her Self. Petrified, she can't respond [...] caught between [...] the different worlds she inhabits.[52]

There is some previous research which resonates with Farah's account, and Anzaldúa's words, in that it hypothesises that difficulties in speaking might arise from social anxiety,[53] or indeed be an extreme manifestation of fear in social situations.[54] This problematises the idea that these diagnoses—SAD, SM—are discrete disease entities reflecting underlying pathology: a notion to which the *DSM-5*'s schema, and the biomedical model which underpins it, subscribes. Rather, these experiences can be rendered comprehensible by exploring the cultural milieu in which they occur.

In order to do this for Farah, I note that she echoes an idea running through the stories of people with SM having to do with others' expectations. Psychologists Aaron S. Walker and Jane Tobbell,[55] in their exploration of the narratives of individuals with SM, discuss 'the expectations of others who had adapted to, and in doing so reinforced, the silence of the child'.[56] Farah spoke about the weight of others' expectations when visiting her home country in Western Asia, and how these caused her to embrace a personality more reminiscent of her past self. '[I]n my mind', she explained to me, 'I have this memory of myself, that I was like that in this environment, so, unconsciously I would be the same again.' She experienced something similar when seeing childhood friends from back home, telling me

> [W]hen I started to visit them again, after years [...] I could see that it was a bit hard for them to see me differently [...] I've changed a lot [...] I try to be... A bit like twenty years ago, when I'm around them.

This facet of Farah's experience might be read through the lens of her lived experience as an immigrant. Writing on the bicultural identity performance of immigrants, Deaux and Greenwood state that '[i]mmigrants live between at least two cultural groups and cultural traditions: those of the host country and those of the country of origin'.[57] Anzaldúa has termed the spaces betwixt two cultures 'borderland spaces',[58] and Deaux and Greenwood put forth that it is within these borderlands that 'immigrants must decide how (and whether) to maintain or transform their identities of origin in tandem with developing new identities anchored in the culture and traditions of the receiving country'.[59] Perhaps then, the recency of Farah's move to the UK from another country was culpable in her speaking difficulties: she had not yet had time to navigate this bifurcation in her identity.

Deaux and Greenwood raise another point salient to Farah's account. That is, the way in which immigrants 'negotiate, perform, or silence their identities'[60] is contingent on the audience. When visiting her home country, Farah is arguably silencing the 'new' identity which she associates with the UK, and trying to perform the 'old' identity to which her friends back home are accustomed. This is reminiscent of how individuals with SM in Walker and Tobell's study 'negotiated their identities with regards [*sic*] to the expectations and behaviours of others'.[61] Indeed, feeling as though they would be 'unable to handle the reactions of others if they were to suddenly begin [*sic*] speaking' was cited as a reason for the perpetuation of SM in Walker and Tobell's work.[62]

Scott cites a similar explanation for the perpetuation of the shy identity in writing that 'it may be easier for a person to live up to the label they have been given than to try and change the opinions of others'.[63] Farah hinted at this in telling me about her friends' reactions upon seeing how she had changed: 'I could see that it was a bit uncomfortable for them.' To explore exactly why Farah might have performed her 'old' identity in a bid not to make her childhood friends uncomfortable, I wish to cite a remark made by Amy, who told me that her own 'social anxiety is probably tied to what I have been programmed to think, as a woman [...] that my responsibility is to make other people comfortable'. Building on Amy's words, just as being unable to handle others' reactions keeps individuals with SM silent, the need to make others *comfortable* constrains the behaviours that socially anxious women exhibit. This is especially the case when these behaviours contravene gendered norms, as Farah explained: 'I've changed a lot [...] the way that I insist on what I want [...] and what is wrong, what is bad.'

Having discussed ASD and SM, I now want to address a further diagnosis which is listed as being 'co-morbid' with SAD by the *DSM-5*:

Avoidant Personality Disorder (APD).[64] Like Neurodevelopmental Disorders, 'Personality Disorders' are somewhat distinct from other psychiatric diagnoses but are still within psychiatry's remit. A Personality Disorder is defined as

> [A]n enduring pattern of inner experience and behavior that *deviates markedly from the expectations of the individual's culture*, is pervasive and inflexible, has an onset in adolescence or early adulthood, is stable over time, and leads to distress or impairment.[65]

Behaviours which challenge cultural ideals, and their pathologisation, therefore seem to be an integral part of Personality Disorders.

APD in particular is described as 'a pattern of social inhibition, feelings of inadequacy, and hypersensitivity to negative evaluation'.[66] Although none of the participants mentioned this diagnosis explicitly, a number of their sentiments evoked it in that they described 'feelings of inadequacy'[67] and 'low self-esteem'.[68] Daniella told me that, since being 'six or seven', she 'would always have this feeling of being inadequate [...] inferior to everyone else'. These feelings persisted throughout her teenage years, right through to when she graduated from a respected university with an upper-second class honours degree. She downplayed this accomplishment, instead communicating that she 'did alright'. Farah also alluded to feelings of inadequacy in sharing with me how she had won a highly competitive scholarship to study at her university. She said of the awarding panel: 'I still think that they didn't realise that I'm not good.' Similarly, Amy divulged that, in the context of her academic research, she believed she was 'probably fooling everybody else [...] fewer people are working on that so they won't know that it's all a lie'.

That these attitudes featured so prominently in these women's narratives muddies the waters between 'APD' and 'SAD', a muddying to which even the *DSM-5* concedes: there is 'a great deal of overlap between avoidant personality disorder and social anxiety disorder (social phobia), so much so that they may be alternative conceptualizations of the same or similar conditions',[69] or indeed on the same 'spectrum'.[70] Likewise, Robert Spitzer, who led the task force which updated the *DSM* to form its third edition, describes 'almost "total overlap"'[71] between the two diagnoses. Even Michael Liebowitz, who was one of the pioneering researchers on SAD, has said that 'it doesn't make sense to have these two separate categories'.[72]

This lack of distinction is a prime example of why Carl I. Cohen is so critical of the *DSM*'s alleged objective cataloguing of 'disease entities'.[73] While I am writing on the poor demarcation between these 'disorders', my stance is not revisionist. My contention is that these poorly defined diagnoses are a *reflection*, a *symptom* of the notion I am arguing against in this book. That is, the notion that these diagnoses are discrete disease entities which are caused by biological malfunction. Rather, the slippage between them exposes the fact that they are arbitrary, subjective categories which have been created to pathologise non-normativity.

As I talked to participants, it became increasingly clear that several of them did not seem to subscribe to the *DSM-5*'s conception of diagnoses as separate illnesses either. Rather, they viewed their different experiences of distress—or, in psychiatric terms, diagnoses—as interlocking and without clear boundaries. In speaking about sadness—which the *DSM-5* would term 'Major Depressive Disorder'—Amy described how her emotional states 'kind of bounce off of each other':

> My logic brain is going, 'Hey, you seem like you're in a depression rut. The main thing you could do to help get out of that would be to reach out to your friends.' [...] But my social anxiety goes, 'What if a depressed person is not a palatable person to hang out with?'

Amy's account describes social anxiety and sadness as mutually reinforcing. In feeling sad, she is uneasy about interacting with others; her isolation then deepens her unhappiness. Phoebe also challenged the psy sciences' conception of neatly separated disease entities in characterising her varied experiences of mental distress thus: '[T]hey all like kind of blur into one, don't they? [...] you don't know which is which, often.'

This way of viewing one's mental distress could also suggest why a number of the women I interviewed had not sought help for social anxiety specifically: perhaps they did not view SAD as distinct. On this point, the *ICD-10* defines 'Generalised Anxiety Disorder' (GAD) as '[a]nxiety that is generalized and persistent but not restricted to, or even strongly predominating in, any particular environmental circumstances (i.e. it is "free-floating")'.[74] But if feelings of nervousness pervade all areas of life, and are equally distressing in social situations as in other areas, then cleaving this nervousness into 'GAD' and 'SAD' seems somewhat arbitrary. What seemed to make more sense was how Phoebe and Amy thought about this distinction: Phoebe identified her different types of mental distress as 'com[ing] under quite a broad umbrella', while Amy called her social anxiety 'the social aspect, the social anxiety sect of generalised anxiety'.

On Amy's remark, the slippage between diagnostic criteria for GAD and SAD is emblematic of the hazy demarcation between diagnoses in broader terms. More to the point, the APA's volume *Anxiety Disorders: DSM-5 Selections*'s criteria for GAD actually *include* some elements which are germane to social anxiety. That is, 'Social worries are common in generalized anxiety disorder, but the focus is more on the nature of ongoing relationships rather than on fear of negative evaluation.'[75] Some of the women in my sample problematised this distinction in that their fear of negative evaluation occurred *within* ongoing relationships:

> Phoebe: I get really anxious about when I see my friends. I will obsess afterwards [...] '[D]o they just not like me anymore?'

> Ellen: [I]f I haven't seen a group of people for a while then I'll be really anxious [...] I'm like, '[...] what are we going to talk about?'

> Olivia: Sometimes I'm absolutely fine around the people I'm close to, but other times I feel anxious [...] worrying about how I am being perceived and [...] if I'm going to ruin the relationship somehow and not meet their expectations of me!

> Amy: [D]inner with my friends [...] my social anxiety, it gets in there and it convinces me that they're just putting in the time because they feel like they have to [...] 'You're annoying people.'

As we are examining the interplay between social anxiety and anxiety more generally, it is worth considering how this might impact women's help-seeking. Viewing social anxiety as a subset of anxiety—as Amy told us—or as coming under the umbrella of mental distress more broadly—as Phoebe said—might create the impression that treatment for one could iron the other out. Olivia articulated this in describing her own help-seeking: 'I was visiting the GP primarily for depression, but since I knew that anxiety is often linked with depression I also mentioned struggling with social anxiety.'

While this could partially explain participants' reluctance to seek help for social anxiety specifically, the narratives of Amy and Olivia suggested another reason. As Farah and Amy had earlier spoken about the mandate that they make others feel comfortable, Amy and Olivia both told me that their gender socialisation demands that they put others' feelings first:

> Amy: [W]omen are more susceptible to Social Anxiety Disorder, probably on the basis that we're conditioned to be more concerned with other people's feelings than our own [...] and that puts the burden of other people's mental states on us [...] it makes every social interaction terrifying, if you walk into it feeling responsible for the feelings and experiences of everyone around you.

> Olivia: I'm always trying to be pleasing and nice and untroublesome and thoughtful of how others might feel or respond to what I've said—traditionally feminine characteristics.

Given this, psychiatrist Siegfried Kasper's description of SAD as 'characteristically discreet',[76] to which he attributes its under-diagnosis, is ironically fitting. While he is writing of its relative invisibility compared with Panic Disorder and GAD, I argue that SAD's being 'discreet' in women is precisely due to its being imbued with norms of femininity. That is, women experience social anxiety because society puts others' feelings in our hands. Our resulting concern with the effect we have on others is therefore *not* a contravention of expected gender norms. In turn, social anxiety is unlikely to be construed as offensive, a disorder, or a medical issue. Hence, it is not likely to be viewed as problematic by others—the same others who persuade women to seek help—because others actually stand to *benefit* from it: women's social anxiety is undergirded by concern for others' emotional wellbeing. As such, while the socially anxious experience, broadly, is considered a sickness, or aberrant, this facet of social anxiety in women is arguably *not deviant* since it accords with expected gender norms.

Like Olivia and Amy, Orbach remarks upon these gender norms. She explains that women are held responsible for others' emotional wellbeing, for we 'grow up to be concerned with others and often feel guilty if we notice that we have our own needs, desires and concerns which really come first'.[77] Paula J. Caplan also speaks to this in describing how women often 'feel guilty because their socialization leads them to believe they are selfish for feeling unhappy or needing help. After all, women are not supposed to want or need anything for themselves'.[78] This source of women's guilt is made more evident by considering the words of author and academic Lisa Downing: for men, being selfish is but a 'minor infraction'; by contrast, '[I]t is a far more serious transgression to be selfish while a woman – indeed it is a category violation of identity.'[79]

Following this, Olivia's and Amy's narratives echo a point made in Chap. 2: that women are expected to be solely responsible for their relationships,[80] and 'not upsetting people must always be given priority'.[81] Indeed, women are expected to carry out the bulk of emotional labour in relationships[82]—something of which Ria was very much aware. She described how 'there's a pressure for women to [...] be primary caregivers [...] even if you don't have children [...] to be the person who sort of holds the social unit or the family unit together'. This evokes sociologists Walter Gove and Michael Hughes's work on the relationship between women's social role and Talcott Parsons's sick role:

> [W]omen in our society are generally expected to occupy a nurturant role, both performing daily the *essential* household tasks and taking on the major responsibility for the care of children, spouses and aged relatives. As a consequence [...] women will find it more difficult than men to adopt the sick role completely.[83]

While this provides further context to participants' unwillingness to seek help, it also flags up a void in their narratives: none of them reported enjoying the 'exemption from normal social role responsibilities'[84] that the sick role is supposed to entail—even when their mental distress was severe, enduring, or both.

The concepts of social roles, gender roles, norms, and normativities have formed a backdrop to this chapter thus far in discussing the significance of 'co-morbidities'—other types of mental distress, neurodiversity—in women's social anxiety. But what other incarnations can these 'co-morbidities' take? To explore this, we must widen our focus and give greater consideration to the body.

Physicality

Amy in particular spoke at length about the interplay between her physicality and her mental distress. Having been born with a heart defect, she told me: '[A] big portion of my mental health is probably tied to the infant trauma that I had when I had the first heart surgeries, when I was born.' Viewing Amy's mental distress as an intelligible response to disturbing experiences calls to mind R. D. Laing's notion that insanity is 'a perfectly rational adjustment to an insane world'.[85] Following Laing, Amy's emotional states—sadness, nervousness—can be thought of as perfectly rational adjustments to, as she described, 'a lifetime of facing mortality'.

In order to cope with this dark prospect, Amy explained that she had engaged in 'therapy [...] in a run up to heart surgery' as a young adult. After the surgery, she described how she expected her mental distress to disappear, but instead found herself thinking, '[M]y brain still doesn't really work though.' As such, 'physical health', she told me, 'gave a tangible reason to investigate my mental health' and 'ended up paving the way for an acknowledgement of my mental health'. Although Amy believed her mental distress to be rooted in childhood trauma related to her heart defect, she also said: '[M]y mental health is its own thing and it's not just a symptom of physical health.' With that said, Amy gave examples of the reverse: namely, the physical manifestations of her mental distress. She explained:

> [A]nxiety affecting your appetite [...] getting physical nausea in an anxiety standpoint [...] in terms of physical symptoms of depression, like physical lethargy is a big one, I tend to get quite cold in that as well [...] just a general slowing kind of melancholic kind of space.

What is significant about Amy's perspective, and what evokes the entanglement of the mental with the physical, is that her mental distress and physical health oftentimes produce the same sensations. On this point, she described to me how she would sometimes find herself wondering,

> '[A]m I palpitating because I have anxiety, or am I palpitating because there's blood physically backed up in my heart as a result of my problematic mechanical valve?' [...] [T]hese [...] tangible, mechanical, anatomical problems having the same symptoms, in some cases, as my less tangible mental health.

Amy's lived experience has thus given her insight into the body's interconnectedness, since 'it makes it difficult to determine which symptoms are coming from which things and sometimes it's both'. Like feminist scholars' writings on gendered psychiatric diagnoses,[86] her narrative suggests that considering the mind and the body separately is unhelpful for fully understanding women's experiences of mental distress. Indeed, Amy emphasises 'the significance of acknowledging that the whole body is interconnected and the psychological stuff affects the physical and vice versa'.

Farah echoed this point, for she related instances in which her social anxiety brought about physical symptoms:

> [M]y heartbeat [...] [i]n a way that I couldn't breathe [...] I'm getting... red [...] So hot [...] I can feel exactly the [...] moving, blood [...] Shaking hands [...] trembling hands! [...] when I get stressed [...] I feel sick [...] sweating.

In a similar vein, Daniella said that her nervousness made her 'feel queasy and nauseous, and dizzy'. Crucially, Daniella proposed that SAD is 'not just, you know, a mental disorder, it's kind of a physical disorder because obviously it affects everything: your body, your blood pressure can go up and your heart rate can go up'. An article by the Royal College of Psychiatrists entitled 'Shyness and social phobia' outlines the interplay between emotions and the body in describing how '[o]ther people may be able to see some of the signs of this anxiety – the blushing, stammering, shaking and trembling'. In turn, 'You worry so much about looking worried that you actually do look worried.'[87] Daniella's narrative evoked the formation of this loop—physical symptoms arising from her emotions then affecting how she feels—in that she told me, 'You actually feel like you're ill inside.'

Ellen's testimony also evoked a loop in that she described her experience with Joint Hypermobility Syndrome:[88]

> I have like chronic joint pain which is linked to the depression and anxiety [...] I'm more prone to injury [...] so then I'm less likely to be able to exercise and then I get anxious [...] it like goes round in circles.

At this point, it is necessary to touch on mind-body dualism, which is still a matter of debate within psychiatry today.[89] The concept has a long history, being closely associated with the work of philosopher René Descartes, beginning in the seventeenth century.[90] Some feminist thinkers, such as Genevieve Lloyd and Moira Gatens,[91] have used the work of philosopher Baruch Spinoza as an alternative way of theorising about the mind and the body. Specifically, they have found his tenets that the mind is 'the idea of the body'[92] and that 'the mind and body are one thing, viewed in two irreducibly different ways'[93] useful insofar as they offer a different paradigm to that espoused by Descartes.[94] As to why this is needed, we can look to some of Laing's remarks which are implicitly critical of Cartesian dualism:

> The most serious objection to the technical vocabulary currently used to describe psychiatric patients is that it consists of words which split man up verbally in a way which is analogous to the existential splits we have to describe here.[95]

Language *itself* therefore places constraints on how we conceptualise and express different aspects of our lived experience: it verbally splits us up into 'mind' and 'body'. Like Laing, Amy was critical of this splitting up:

> [D]on't get me started on the mind-body stuff [...] a huge, huge, huge element of medicine is understanding how this part of the body affects that part of the body, and even down to the split between mental health and physical health. That's a fallacy.

Amy's words are reminiscent of tenets from feminist work on women's mental distress, notably those of Jane M. Ussher on PMS. Ussher argues that women's bodily, social, and psychological levels cannot be disentangled.[96] Likewise, Amy told me that

> It's a fallacy and a human construct of medicine that we think of the body as a series of layered systems that can be separated out from each other. Because you can't [...] the body is a big, messy, organic thing.

Amy's thoughts on inseparability also call to mind Joan C. Chrisler and Ingrid Johnston-Robledo's conceptualisation of the interplay between the body and the self, for they posit that '[w]ithout a body, there is no self [...] a living body provides a home for the self, and the brain creates the mind, which produces the sense of self'.[97] Another way of considering this is by using the concept of embodiment, which, in the words of sociologist Simon J. Williams, offers a means by which we can 'tackle, head on, the traditional division between biology and society, mind and body'.[98] Academic Margot Lyon also advocates abandoning mind-body splits, telling us that instead we must

> [C]onfront the question of how the social realm itself is embodied: a notion which can give form to the relationship between the social structural milieu in which humans live, their subjective experience, and the *flesh* through which that existence is lived.[99]

Most germane to this book's approach, embodiment has been utilised by several feminist thinkers. Drawing on the discipline of cognitive psychology, Chrisler and Johnston-Robledo define embodiment as 'the effect the body has on shaping the mind' and 'the effect of the body on the self'.[100] Moreover, Elizabeth Mollard emphasises that women cannot be divided up into parts,[101] highlighting the inextricability of the biological and the psychological in much the same way as Amy's testimony does.

Participants' descriptions of how their social anxiety manifests physically further illustrate this inextricability. What we can further glean from their narratives is that the biological and psychological have a mutually reinforcing relationship: think about Daniella's alluding to how physical symptoms arising from her emotions affect how she feels—'ill inside'—and Ellen's joint pain constraining the amount of exercise she can do which, in turn, worsens her depression and anxiety. As such, although social anxiety might be, at least in the very first instance, experienced in mental terms, it is thereafter experienced by the woman in her entirety: an embodied experience. Williams makes a related point in underscoring the importance of emotions in life, wherein he describes the body as

> [T]he active, emotionally 'expressive' body, in sickness and in health, as the basis of self, sociality, meaning and order, set within the socio-cultural realms of everyday life and the ritualised forms of interaction and exchange they involve.[102]

A position connected to Williams's is adopted by medical humanities scholar Elizabeth J. Donaldson. She holds that 'theories that pay attention exclusively to the social causes and construction of mad identity while overlooking the material conditions of the body, and the body as a material condition, have a limited political scope'.[103] That several participants highlighted the part that specifically female experiences or constitutions played in their social anxiety provides an apt opportunity to bring Williams's and Donaldson's ideas to bear on this gendered form of mental distress:

> Ria: [W]e do have a hormonal fluctuation sort of in-built into our being as well, and that's a legit thing, isn't it?
>
> Daniella: Hormones play a role in a sense. Because you've got lots of hormones that are fluctuating throughout the… Month.
>
> Ellen: [T]here's definitely points in my like cycle, of the month, as well, that I'm worse.

When Ellen elaborated on this, she hinted that it was not necessarily hormonal changes around menstruation *per se* that affected her mood. Rather, she spoke about how the changes in her body which accompanied these hormonal changes made her feel:

> I was reading, and it was like, 'You can put on up to 5lbs,' and I'm like, 'I am that person that puts that on.' [...] I can't do any of my clothes up when I'm on my period [...] I'm like, 'I hate myself,' and none of my clothes fit.

Ellen is alluding to temporary weight gain having a negative effect on her self-esteem. And although her body *is* a linchpin in this, it is likely that her exposure to the social conditions which mandate women's slenderness is strongly implicated in her mental distress. Ellen's account therefore exemplifies how considering the materiality of the body *in* its sociocultural, and especially gendered, context is necessary to provide a full picture of the socially anxious woman's experience.

Since I am discussing some participants' attributions of their mental distress—at least, in part—to hormonal fluctuations, I must be clear about one thing: my repudiation of biologically reductionist accounts which attribute the heightened prevalence of Depression and Anxiety Disorders in women primarily to their hormonal profiles.[104] With that said, and although my overarching focus *is* on the under-researched social contributors to women's SAD, I am not dismissing the effects of the body. This gives rise to a tension, and it is one with which other scholars have grappled. Literary scholar Catherine Prendergast muses on how to resolve this in the case of schizophrenia:

> For an academic like myself with generally poststructuralist leanings, to think of schizophrenia as a 'disease' makes me sound at best conservative and at worst theoretically unsound. I am therefore left wandering far from my usual terrain to find language with which I can address the dilemmas and gaps in understanding that mental illness presents.[105]

And Ussher elucidates a comparable dilemma in her work on PMS:

> One of the main problems is that in adopting a social constructionist perspective, or in arguing that PMS exists entirely at a discursive level, we are implicitly denying the influence of biology — of factors such as menstruation, hormonal changes, or endocrine changes — or we may appear to relegate the body to a passive subsidiary role, which has meaning or

> interpretation imposed upon it. Whilst the emphasis on social and discursive phenomena is understandable as a reaction against biological reductionism, positioning the body as irrelevant in the etiology, interpretation, or meaning of PMS or premenstrual symptomatology is clearly inappropriate.[106]

As such, although my focus on social contributors to women's SAD *is*, in part, a response to biological reductionism, it is a *focus*, not an exclusive consideration. It does not preclude considering the body—rather, the holistic perspective outlined in the previous chapter *requires* considering the body. Ellen perhaps best sums up the approach to be taken here in saying: '[Y]es, I can be a bit more anxious on my period, but also, I'm mostly more anxious because of the way that men have spoken to me, in the past.'

To further outline the importance of the body in women's SAD, I would like to bring in the thoughts of feminist science and technology studies scholar Donna Haraway while revisiting the work of Spinoza. Haraway tells us that 'bodies are perfectly "real," and [...] corporealization is tropic and historically specific at every layer of its tissues'.[107] Likewise, Gatens relays Spinoza's point that the body is 'not identical with itself across time', for 'its meaning and capacities will vary according to its context'[108] and 'can only be revealed by the ongoing interactions of the body and its environment'.[109] This latter point is key, since it is through interacting with the environment, and the people in it, that social anxiety is experienced. In the same vein, Donaldson endorses the idea that 'bodies are not simply born, but made'.[110] And Haraway tells us that 'bodies as subjects of knowledge are material-semiotic generative nodes. Their boundaries materialize in social interactions; "objects" like bodies do not pre-exist as such'.[111] To take the liberty of appropriating Simone de Beauvoir's famous remark for my own purposes:[112] 'One is not born, but rather becomes, a socially anxious woman.'

Haraway's remark on how social interaction shapes the body is crucial to an analysis of social anxiety, and this was something which arose in my conversation with Ria. Ria is a highly capable British-Punjabi woman who works as a scientist in a male-dominated field. As she sat across from me and we sipped our coffee, I recall being struck by how erudite and articulate she was. But in spite of her brilliance and fierce intellect, I was saddened, and angered, by her experiences of being undermined, patronised, and underestimated in the workplace. Her stories likely also struck a chord with me because, since I had previously used my undergraduate degree in

Physics and worked in this field, her anecdotes seemed all too familiar. After having described but a few incidents to me, Ria resignedly said, '[W]hen it happens more than once and you're aware of it [...] eventually, it's going to chip away at you, isn't it?'

The 'chipping away' to which Ria alludes has much in common with 'microaggressions'. Ria's testimony suggests that our reaction to outside stimuli, namely repeated unfair treatment in the form of these microaggressions, causes negative emotions and, by virtue of these emotions being rooted in our brains, they are rooted in our bodies. Williams phrases this another way in observing that 'society affects us, both emotionally and physically, deep within the recesses of the human body'.[113] Ria spoke on this point in pondering the origins of social anxiety:

> [I]nstinctually, I'd sort of say the social/environmental would be the sort of, the base of it [...] Biology obviously is a thing, but yeah, it's kind of carefully cultivated, isn't it? Maybe due to a mix of all these biologies coming together [...] I think it is the result of lots of little interactions building up over time [...] a lone instance that suddenly makes you socially anxious: I don't think that's a thing.

She continued by saying that

> [W]ider culture can be a thing. I think experiences of being sort of talked down to don't help, along with an idea that [...] maybe, in some senses, you're inferior. So sort of having a general impression that's reinforced by specific experience.

This segment of Ria's testimony is reminiscent of Anzaldúa's exposition of *la facultad*. *La facultad* is 'the capacity to see in surface phenomena the meaning of deeper realities, to see the deep structure below the surface'.[114] Further to this, Anzaldúa relates that '[t]hose who are pushed out of the tribe for being different are likely to become more sensitized' in this phenomenon.[115] This resonates with another of Ria's remarks, for she told me, '[Y]ou sort of feel a sense of your lack of worth being reinforced with little things—*sometimes possibly very little things.*'[116] It was not only Ria who alluded to having heightened sensitivity to surface phenomena which reflect deeper structural inequalities. Farah also indicated that she experienced this in telling me, 'Sometimes you feel like you just fight for some basic things... That it's not fair [...] but if you share it then people say,

"Well, you're so sensitive."' Anzaldúa notes that *la facultad* is strongest in '[t]hose who do not feel psychologically or physically safe in the world [...] the females, the homosexuals of all races, the darkskinned, the outcast, the persecuted, the marginalized, the foreign'.[117] It is perhaps then not coincidental that it was in the narratives of Ria and Farah—both multiply burdened as women of colour and, in Farah's case, as an immigrant—that I found strongest resonance with *la facultad*.

Relating the surface phenomena of *la facultad* in the environment, which can be found in the form of microaggressions, to our biology, Ria earlier mentioned 'careful cultivation'. This could be interpreted as repeated social interactions of a similar kind having effects on our emotions and, by extension, our bodies. Sue gives a relevant anecdote about a time when he, an Asian American man, and his colleague, an African American woman, both felt discriminated against because of their race. At the time, Sue recalled asking himself, '[W]hy were we being singled out? Were we being singled out because of our race? Was this just a random event with no racial overtones? Were we being oversensitive and petty?'[118] After the incident in question, Sue and his colleague both 'felt resentment, irritation, and anger'.[119] And as Ria alluded to emotional states, which arise from experiencing microaggressions, having an effect on our biology, Sue's account continues as follows: 'While I kept telling myself to drop the matter, I could feel my blood pressure rising, my heart beating faster, and my face flushing with anger.'[120] In the spirit of both Spinoza's account of the body and Haraway's work, we are beginning to see how the body of the socially anxious woman is made.[121]

In attempting to reconcile the mind-body split in the case of the socially anxious woman, I found myself contemplating other splits and how they relate to one another. Gatens has spoken about this in her interview with philosopher Susan James. Therein, she shares how she first began reading Spinoza because she was interested in the mind-body problem 'and its relation to the reason/passion split and *the nature/culture split*'.[122] Williams likewise describes how the mind/body split 'spawns a number of other dualisms such as *nature/culture*, reason/emotion, public/private'.[123] Navigating the nature-culture dualism was a recurring theme when participants speculated about the origins of their SAD:

> Daniella: [T]he way you're brought up, has an effect [...] I think it depends [...] on your personality as well, so it's nature and nurture.

> Amy: It's sort of the nature vs. nurture question, isn't it, at a certain point? [...] our experiences are a bit of both.

> Olivia: I think what 'causes' SAD may be a combination of predisposition to social anxiety in genetics and personality, mixed with environmental and social upbringing within cultural norms of gender/femininity. The contributing factors for me were a mixture of nature and nurture.

These narratives all regard culture *and* biology as having a bearing on social anxiety. Gatens develops this in citing traditional political theory which 'takes the body [...] as virtually given'.[124] That is, the way that the body 'takes up' culture is contingent on this *a priori* biology. This traditional viewpoint was present in Amy's narrative, for she told me that 'having a mental illness is genuinely a condition of chemical imbalances. So that's an internal space that could then be exacerbated by external influences'.

Gatens however *departs* from this traditional viewpoint in advocating for a 'nondichotomized view of nature and culture' which, in a nod to Haraway's earlier cited tenet, requires 'acknowledging the cultural and historical specificity of bodies'.[125] In other words, '[T]he body is *always already* in a social context.'[126] Phoebe's musings on the evolution of social anxiety echoed this, for she remarked: '[T]he way in which society is structured massively has an impact on our brains [...] you can't ever like remove yourself from those structures, because it's kind of what shape[s] us.' Olivia's words also resonated with Gatens's thoughts, for she told me:

> I think I'm predisposed to be on the quiet and shy side, and feminine cultural norms only cemented these traits and boxed me in rather than nurture me to feel more empowered [...] It's very difficult to untangle yourself from sociocultural norms and beliefs about gender.

Most pertinent to Olivia's narrative, Gatens contends that 'the context in which a body grows makes a real difference to the powers and capacities of the individual it becomes'.[127]

As such, eschewing a bifurcated view of nature and culture—and other, associated splits, such as mind and body—gives insight into how the socially anxious woman is born. Crucially, this point of view allows for considering the significance of the body without resorting to biological reductionism which presents mental distress as innate and individual.

Rather, delving into the interrelation between the environment and biology results in a holistic examination of how harmful societal conditions can give rise to social anxiety in women.

Notes

1. Talcott Parsons, *The Social System* (New York and Toronto: The Free Press, 1964), p. 437.
2. Ibid., p. 430.
3. Matthias Zick Varul, 'Talcott Parsons, the Sick Role and Chronic Illness', *Body & Society*, 16.2 (2010), 72–94 https://doi.org/10.1177/1357034X10364766 p. 75.
4. Parsons, *The Social System*, p. 475.
5. Eliot Freidson, 'Client Control and Medical Practice', *American Journal of Sociology*, 65.4 (1960), 374–82 https://doi.org/10.1086/222726
6. Susie Orbach and Luise Eichenbaum, *Understanding Women* (Harmondsworth: Penguin, 1985), p. 7.
7. Katie Masters, 'Women's Experiences of Social Anxiety Disorder: Privileging Marginalised Perspectives and Rewriting Dominant Narratives', *International Mad Studies Journal*, 1.1 (2022), e1–21 https://doi.org/10.58544/imsj.v1i1.5244
8. Ibid.
9. Parsons, *The Social System*, p. 437.
10. Ibid., p. 285.
11. Barbara Louise Blackwell, 'Upper Middle Class Adult Expectations about Entering the Sick Role for Physical and Psychiatric Dysfunctions', *Journal of Health and Social Behavior*, 8.2 (1967), 83–95 https://doi.org/10.2307/2948339 p. 95.
12. J. Twardowski, *5 Ways To Care for Yourself during your Menstruation* (2015) http://jennifertwardowski.com/2015/04/13/5-ways-to-care-foryourself-during-your-menstruation/ cited in Molly McKinney, 'Sick Bodies in Healthcare Culture: Health Communication that Disciplines Female Bodies', in *Transgressing Feminist Theory and Discourse: Advancing Conversations across Disciplines*, ed. by Jimmie Manning and Jennifer C. Dunn (London: Routledge, 2018).
13. American Psychiatric Association, *Diagnostic and Statistical Manual of Mental Disorders* [*DSM-5*] (Washington, DC: American Psychiatric Association Publishing, 2013) https://ebookcentral.proquest.com/lib/bham/reader.action?docID=1811753 [accessed 6 January 2021] p. 208.
14. Lennard J. Davis, *Enforcing Normalcy: Disability, Deafness, and the Body* (London and New York: Verso, 1995), p. 29.

15. Albert Camus, *The Stranger* [*L'Étran*ger] trans. Matthew Ward (New York: Vintage International, 1989 [1942]), p. 37.
16. Judi Chamberlin, *On Our Own: Patient-controlled Alternatives to the Mental Health System* (Lawrence, Massachusetts: National Empowerment Centre, Inc., 2012[1977]), p. 229.
17. Ibid., p. 211.
18. A diagnosis of Social Anxiety Disorder is not likely to be grounds for detention under the Mental Health Act, the criterion for which is that the individual 'need[s] urgent treatment for a mental health disorder and [is] at risk of harm to themselves or others'. See NHS, *Mental Health Act* (2022) https://www.nhs.uk/mental-health/social-care-and-your-rights/mental-health-and-the-law/mental-health-act/ [accessed 11 January 2023].
19. Chamberlin, *On Our Own*, p. 71.
20. Ibid.
21. Ibid., p. 186.
22. E.g. Ronald David Laing, quoted in Larry Chang, *Wisdom for the Soul: Five Millennia of Prescriptions for Spiritual Healing* (Washington DC: Gnosophia Publishing, 2006), p. 412.
    Ronald David Laing, *The Divided Self: An Existential Study in Sanity and Madness* (London: Tavistock Publications Ltd., 1965).
    David Cooper, *Psychiatry and Anti-psychiatry*, 2nd edn (St. Albans: Paladin, 1972).
23. Davis, *Enforcing Normalcy*, p. 163.
24. Tom Shakespeare, 'The Social Model of Disability', in *The Disability Studies Reader*, ed. by Lennard J. Davis, 4th edn (London and New York: Routledge, 2013), 214–21, p. 216.
25. Anita Thapar, Miriam Cooper, and Michael Rutter, 'Neurodevelopmental Disorders', *The Lancet Psychiatry*, 4.4 (2017), 339–46 https://doi.org/10.1016/S2215-0366(16)30376-5
26. Courtenay Frazier Norbury and Alison Sparks, 'Difference or Disorder? Cultural Issues in Understanding Neurodevelopmental Disorders', *Developmental Psychology*, 49.1 (2013), 45–58 https://doi.org/10.1037/a0027446 cited in Erika Dyck and Ginny Russell, 'Challenging Psychiatric Classification: Healthy Autistic Diversity and the Neurodiversity Movement', in *Healthy Minds in the Twentieth Century: In and beyond the Asylum*, ed. by Steven J. Taylor and Alice Brumby (Cham, Switzerland: Palgrave Macmillan, 2020), 167–87, p. 172.
27. APA, *DSM-5*, p. 50.
28. WHO, 'Pervasive Developmental Disorders', *ICD-10* (2016) https://icd.who.int/browse10/2016/en#/F84 [accessed 7 January 2021].

29. National Autistic Society, *Professionals Involved in a Diagnosis* (2020) https://www.autism.org.uk/about/diagnosis/professionals-involved.aspx [accessed 24 September 2020].
30. Dyck and Russell, 'Challenging Psychiatric Classification', p. 171.
31. Davis, *Enforcing Normalcy*, p. xv.
32. Ibid., p. 7.
33. Dyck and Russell, 'Challenging Psychiatric Classification', p. 176.
34. Jim Sinclair, 'Don't Mourn for Us', *Autonomy, The Journal of Critical Autism Studies*, 1.1 (2012), 1–4 https://philosophy.ucsc.edu/SinclairDontMournForUs.pdf [accessed 16 June 2023] p. 1.
    This extends to linguistic debates within the autism community, which have drawn attention to the *DSM*'s focus on a person 'with ASD', which presents autism as an illness. Instead, identity-first language, such as being 'on the autism spectrum', is proposed as an alternative, since it emphasises neurological variation rather than illness. For more on this, see Kristen Bottema-Beutel, Steven K. Kapp, Jessica Nina Lester, Noah J. Sasson, and Brittany N. Hand, 'Avoiding Ableist Language: Suggestions for Autism Researchers', *Autism in Adulthood* (2021), 18–29 https://doi.org/10.1089/aut.2020.0014
35. APA, *DSM-5*, p. 58.
36. Ibid., pp. 58–59.
37. Derald Wing Sue, *Microaggressions in Everyday Life: Race, Gender, and Sexual Orientation* (John Wiley and Sons Incorporated, 2010) https://ebookcentral.proquest.com/lib/bham/reader.action?docID=487711 [accessed 24 September 2020] p. 45.
38. Jean Piaget, *Language and Thought of the Child (and other Later Works)* (Abingdon: Kegan Paul, 1926).
    Susan Isaacs, *The Nursery Years* (Abingdon: Routledge, 1929).
    All cited in Marion Milner, *A Life of One's Own* (Taylor and Francis Group, 2011) https://ebookcentral.proquest.com/lib/bham/reader.action?docID=672403 [accessed 24 September 2020] p. 84.
39. Milner, *A Life of One's Own*, p. 85.
40. Sue, *Microaggressions*, p. xv.
41. H. Rubin, *Sexism* (2008) http://www.portfolio.com/executives/features/2008/03/17/Sexism-in-the-Workplace? [accessed 19 May 2009].
    Derald Wing Sue and David Sue, *Counseling the Culturally Diverse: Theory and Practice*, 4*th* edn (New York: John Wiley and Sons, 2008).
    US Bureau of the Census, *Poverty in the United States* (Washington, DC: US Government Printing Office, 2002).
    All cited in Sue, *Microaggressions*, p. 164.
42. Sue, *Microaggressions*, p. 164.

43. John F. Dovidio and Samuel L. Gaertner, 'Aversive Racism and Selective Decisions: 1989–1999', *Psychological Science*, 11.4 (2000), 315–19 https://doi.org/10.1111/1467-9280.00262 cited in Sue, *Microaggressions*, p. 54.
44. Sue, *Microaggressions*, p. 54.
45. Ibid., p. 29.
46. Kay Deaux and Ronni Michelle Greenwood, 'Crossing Borders: Intersectional Excursions into Gender and Immigration', in *The SAGE Handbook of Gender and Psychology*, ed. by M. K. Ryan and N. R. Branscombepp (London: Sage Publications, 2013), 234–50, p. 241.
47. Gloria Anzaldúa, *Borderlands La Frontera: The New Mestiza* (San Francisco, CA: Aunt Lute Books, 1987), p. ix.
48. In the case of children only. See APA, *DSM-5*, p. 208.
49. NHS, *Signs of Autism in Adults* (2019) https://www.nhs.uk/conditions/autism/signs/adults/ [accessed 24 September 2020].
50. Also in the case of children only. See APA, *DSM-5*, p. 208.
51. It is worth noting that the example which Farah gave related to recently moving to the UK from another country, so language competence *may* have comprised part of her difficulties. While the *DSM-5* states that such difficulties *do not* constitute an SM diagnosis, they do not seem to be the whole story in Farah's case: the attendant physical manifestations of social anxiety which she describes, as well as the degree to which her account resonates with Anzaldúa's words, cannot be ignored.
52. Anzaldúa, *Borderlands*, p. 20.
53. Bruce Black and Thomas W. Uhde, 'Psychiatric Characteristics of Children with Selective Mutism: A Pilot Study', *Journal of the American Academy of Child and Adolescent Psychiatry*, 34.7 (1995), 847–56 https://doi.org/10.1097/00004583-199507000-00007
    E. Steven Dummit III, Rachel G. Klein, Nancy K. Tancer, Barbara Asche, Jacqueline Martin, and Janet A. Fairbanks, 'Systematic Assessment of 50 Children with Selective Mutism', *Journal of the American Academy of Child and Adolescent Psychiatry*, 36. 5 (1997), 653–60 https://doi.org/10.1097/00004583-199705000-00016
    All cited in Aaron S. Walker and Jane Tobbell, 'Lost Voices and Unlived Lives: Exploring Adults' Experiences of Selective Mutism Using Interpretative Phenomenological Analysis', *Qualitative Research in Psychology*, 12.4 (2015), 453–71 https://doi.org/10.1080/14780887.2015.1054533 p. 453.
54. Josh M. Cisler, Bunmi O. Olatunji, Matthew T. Feldner, and John P. Forsyth, 'Emotion Regulation and the Anxiety Disorders: An Integrative Review', *Journal of Psychopathology and Behavioural Assessment*, 32.1 (2010), 68–82 https://doi.org/10.1007/s10862-009-9161-1

Samantha Scott and Deborah C. Beidel, 'Selective Mutism: An Update and Suggestions for Future Research', *Current Psychiatry Reports*, 13.4 (2011), 251–57 https://doi.org/10.1007/s11920-011-0201-7
All cited in Walker and Tobbell, 'Lost Voices and Unlived Lives', p. 453.
55. Walker and Tobbell, 'Lost Voices and Unlived Lives', p. 456.
56. Ibid.
57. S. Wiley and K. Deaux, 'The Bicultural Identity Performance of Immigrants', in *Identity and Participation in Culturally Diverse Societies*, ed. by A. E. Azzi, X. Chryssochoou, B. Klandermans, and B. Simon (Oxford: Wiley-Blackwell, 2010), 49–68, cited in Deaux and Greenwood, 'Crossing Borders', p. 243.
58. Anzaldúa, *Borderlands*, p. 100.
59. Deaux and Greenwood, 'Crossing Borders', p. 243.
60. Ibid., p. 244.
61. Walker and Tobbell, 'Lost Voices and Unlived Lives', p. 461.
62. Heidi Omdal and David Galloway, 'Interviews with Selectively Mute Children', *Emotional and Behavioural Difficulties*, 12.3 (2007), 205–14 https://doi.org/10.1080/13632750701489956 cited in Walker and Tobbell, 'Lost Voices and Unlived Lives', pp. 462–63.
63. Susie Scott, 'The Shell, the Stranger and the Competent Other: Towards a Sociology of Shyness', *Sociology*, 38.1 (2004), 121–37 https://doi.org/10.1177/0038038504039364 p. 133.
64. APA, *DSM-5*, p. 208.
65. Ibid., p. 645. My emphasis.
66. Ibid.
67. APA, *DSM-5*, p. 673.
68. Ibid.
69. Ibid., p 674.
70. Ibid., p. 648.
71. Robert L. Spitzer, interview by Christopher Lane, 22 February 2006, cited in Christopher Lane, *Shyness: How Normal Behavior Became a Sickness* (Yale University Press, 2007) https://ebookcentral.proquest.com/lib/bham/reader.action?docID=3420940 [accessed 6 January 2021] p. 96.
72. Lane, *Shyness*, pp. 96–97.
73. Carl I. Cohen, 'The Biomedicalization of Psychiatry: A Critical Overview', *Community Mental Health Journal*, 29.6 (1993), 509–21 https://doi.org/10.1007/BF00754260 p. 518.
74. World Health Organization [WHO], 'Social Phobias', *International Classification of Diseases*, 10*th* edn [*ICD-10*] (2016) https://icd.who.int/browse10/2016/en#/F40.1 [accessed 25 September 2020].
75. APA, *Anxiety Disorders: DSM-5 Selections* (Arlington, VA: American Psychiatric Association Publishing, 2016), p. 22.

76. Siegfried Kasper, 'Anxiety Disorders: Under-diagnosed and Insufficiently Treated', *International Journal of Psychiatry in Clinical Practice*, 10.1 (2006), 3–9 https://doi.org/10.1080/13651500600552297 p. 3.
77. Susie Orbach, *Fat Is a Feminist Issue* (London: Arrow Books Limited, 1986), p. 88.
78. Paula J. Caplan, *The Myth of Women's Masochism* (Lincoln, Nebraska: iUniverse, 2005), p. xiv.
79. Lisa Downing, *Selfish Women* (Abingdon, Oxon; New York, NY: Routledge, 2019), p. 1.
80. Dana Crowley Jack, *Silencing the Self: Women and Depression* (Cambridge, MA: Harvard University Press, 1991).
    Helen O'Grady, *Woman's Relationship with Herself: Gender, Foucault, Therapy* (London: Routledge, 2005).
    All cited in Jane M. Ussher and Janette Perz, 'PMS as a Gendered Illness Linked to the Construction and Relational Experience of Hetero-femininity', *Sex Roles*, 68 (2013), 132–50 https://doi.org/10.1007/s11199-011-9977-5 p. 136.
81. Jean Grimshaw, *Philosophy and Feminist Thinking* (Minneapolis: University of Minnesota Press, 1986), p. 196.
82. Jack, *Silencing the Self: Women and Depression.*
    O'Grady, *Woman's Relationship with Herself.*
    All cited in Ussher and Perz, 'PMS as a Gendered Illness', p. 136.
83. Walter R. Gove and Michael Hughes, 'Beliefs vs. Data: More on the Illness Behavior of Men and Women', *American Sociological Review*, 46. 1 (1981), 123–28 https://doi.org/10.2307/2095032 pp. 124, 136, cited in Walter R. Gove, 'Gender Differences in Mental and Physical Illness: The Effects of Fixed Roles and Nurturant Roles', *Social Science & Medicine*, 19.2 (1984), 77–84 https://doi.org/10.1016/0277-9536(84)90273-9 p. 80.
84. Parsons, *The Social System*, p. 437.
85. Laing, quoted in Chang, *Wisdom for the Soul*, p. 412.
86. Jane M. Ussher, 'Premenstrual Syndrome: Reconciling Disciplinary Divides through the Adoption of a Material-discursive Epistemological Standpoint', *Annual Review of Sex Research*, 7.1 (1996), 218–51 https://doi.org/10.1080/10532528.1996.10559914 p. 244.
    Margaret Jane Radin, 'The Pragmatist and the Feminist', *Southern California Law Review*, 63 (1989), 1699–855 https://heinonline.org/HOL/LandingPage?handle=hein.journals/scal63&div=47&id=&page= [accessed 5 January 2021].
    Elizabeth Mollard, 'Exploring Paradigms in Postpartum Depression Research: The Need for Feminist Pragmatism', *Health Care for Women International*, 36.4 (2015), 378–91 https://doi.org/10.1080/07399332.2014.903951 pp. 383, 388.

87. Royal College of Psychiatrists, 'Shyness and Social Phobia', https://www.rcpsych.ac.uk/mental-health/problems-disorders/shyness-and-social-phobia [accessed 6 September 2019].
88. The NHS states: 'Joint hypermobility syndrome is when you have very flexible joints and it causes you pain (you may think of yourself as being double-jointed).' For further information, see NHS, *Joint Hypermobility Syndrome* (2023) https://www.nhs.uk/conditions/joint-hypermobility-syndrome/ [accessed 10 October 2023].
89. Hane Htut Maung, 'Dualism and its Place in a Philosophical Structure for Psychiatry', *Medicine, Health Care and Philosophy*, 22.1 (2019), 59–69 https://doi.org/10.1007/s11019-018-9841-2
    Florence Thibaut, 'The Mind-body Cartesian Dualism and Psychiatry', *Dialogues in Clinical Neuroscience*, 20.1 (2018), 3 https://www.ncbi.nlm.nih.gov/pmc/articles/PMC6016047/ [accessed 25 Septepmber 2020].
    Joachim Raese, 'The Pernicious Effect of Mind/Body Dualism in Psychiatry', *Journal of Psychiatry*, 18.1 (2015), 219–26 https://doi.org/10.4172/1994-8220.1000219
90. René Descartes, *The Philosophical Writing of René Descartes. 3 Vols*, trans. J. Cottingham, R. Stoohoff, D. Murdoch, and A. Kenny (Cambridge, UK: Cambridge University Press, 1984–1991).
    Justin Skirry, *Descartes and the Metaphysics of Human Nature* (London and New York: Thoemmes-Continuum Press, 2005).
    All cited in Thibaut, 'The Mind-body Cartesian Dualism', p. 3.
91. Susan James interviews Genevieve Lloyd and Moira Gatens, 'The Power of Spinoza: Feminist Conjunctions', *Hypatia – Going Australian: Reconfiguring Feminism and Philosophy*, 15.2 (2000), 40–58 https://doi.org/10.1111/j.1527-2001.2000.tb00313.x p. 41.
92. Ibid.
93. Ibid., p. 47.
94. Ibid., p. 41.
95. Laing, *The Divided Self*, p. 19.
96. Ussher, 'Premenstrual Syndrome: Reconciling Disciplinary Divides', p. 244.
97. Joan C. Chrisler and Ingrid Johnston-Robledo, 'Woman's Embodied Self: An Introduction', in *Woman's Embodied Self: Feminist Perspectives on Identity and Image*, ed. by J. C. Chrisler & I. Johnston-Robledo (Washington, DC: American Psychological Association, 2018), 3–14, p. 4.
98. Simon J. Williams, 'Reason, Emotion and Embodiment: Is "Mental" Health a Contradiction in Terms?', *Sociology of Health and Illness*, 22.5 (2000), 559–81 https://doi.org/10.1111/1467-9566.00220 p. 565.

99. Margot Lyon, 'C. Wright Mills Meets Prozac: The Relevance of "Social Emotion" to the Sociology of Health and Illness', *Health and the Sociology of Emotions*, ed. by Veronica James and Jonathan Gabe (Oxford: Blackwell, 1996), 55–78, p. 96.
100. Chrisler and Johnston-Robledo, 'Woman's Embodied Self', p. 8.
101. Elizabeth Mollard, 'Exploring Paradigms in Postpartum Depression Research', pp. 383, 388.
102. Williams, 'Reason, Emotion and Embodiment', p. 567.
103. Elizabeth J. Donaldson, 'The Corpus of the Madwoman: Toward a Feminist Disability Studies Theory of Embodiment and Mental Illness', *National Women's Studies Association Journal*, 14.3 (2002), 99–119 http://www.jstor.org/stable/4316926 [accessed 11 July 2023] p. 102.
104. Katie Masters, 'Tending to the "Neglected Anxiety Disorder": A Critique of the Psy Science Literature on Women and Social Anxiety Disorder', on the panel 'Alternative Perspectives: Humanities Methodologies within Science and Technology Studies', *Nordic Science and Technology Studies Conference 2019*, University of Tampere, 13–14 June 2019.
105. Catherine Prendergast, 'On the Rhetorics of Mental Disability', in *Embodied Rhetorics: Disability in Language and Culture*, ed. by James C. Wilson and Cynthia Lewiecki-Wilson (Carbondale: Southern Illinois University Press, 2001), 45–60, p. 46.
106. Ussher, 'Premenstrual Syndrome: Reconciling Disciplinary Divides', p. 238.
107. Donna Haraway, *Modest_Witness@Second_Millennium. FemaleMan_Meets_OncoMouse: Feminism and Technoscience* (New York: Routledge, 1997), p. 142.
108. Moira Gatens, 'Towards a Feminist Philosophy of the Body', in *Continental Feminism Reader*, ed. by Ann J. Cahill, and Jennifer Hansen (Lanham, Maryland: Rowman and Littlefield, 2003), 275–86, p. 284.
109. Ibid.
110. Donaldson, 'The Corpus of the Madwoman', p. 112.
111. Donna Haraway, 'The Biopolitics of Postmodern Bodies: Determinations of Self in Immune System Discourse', in *Feminist Theory and the Body: A Reader*, ed. by Janet Price and Margrit Shildrick (New York: Routledge, 1999), 203–14, p. 208.
112. Simone de Beauvoir, *The Second Sex* (New York: Vintage Books, 1973), p. 301.
113. Williams, 'Reason, Emotion and Embodiment', p. 569.
114. Anzaldúa, *Borderlands*, p. 38.
115. Ibid.
116. My emphasis.
117. Ibid.

118. Derald Wing Sue, Christina M. Capodilupo, Gina C. Torino, Jennifer M. Bucceri, Aisha M. B. Holder, Kevin L. Nadal, and Marta Esquilin, 'Racial Microaggressions in Everyday Life: Implications for Clinical Practice', *American Psychologist*, 62.4 (2007), 271–86 https://doi.org/10.1037/0003-066X.62.4.271 p. 275.
119. Sue, *Microaggressions*, p. 43.
120. Ibid.
121. Donaldson, 'The Corpus of the Madwoman', p. 112.
122. James interviews Lloyd and Gatens, 'The Power of Spinoza', p. 43. My emphasis.
123. Williams, 'Reason, Emotion and Embodiment', p. 561. My emphasis.
124. Gatens, 'Towards a Feminist Philosophy', p. 284.
125. Ibid.
126. James interviews Lloyd and Gatens, 'The Power of Spinoza', p. 47. My emphasis.
127. Gatens, 'Towards a Feminist Philosophy', p. 284.

CHAPTER 4

Diagnosis, Treatment, and Contingency on (Gendered) Culture

While the previous chapter's opening concerned itself with participants' experiences of help-seeking, this chapter begins by looking at their experiences of what often followed: diagnosis and treatment. When it came to their views on the utility of diagnosis, their opinions were nuanced, and sometimes divergent: some embraced the 'mental illness' label while others rejected it outright. With regard to treatment, those who had been able to access therapy tended to speak of it in positive terms. The consensus on antidepressants, however, was far less clear. But what the women's narratives *did* have in common was a thoughtful conceptualisation of SAD: they all eruditely expressed what 'social anxiety' meant to them. As to whether it warrants treatment, be that with therapy or pharmaceuticals, their accounts evoked the contingency of SAD's classification as a 'mental disorder' on culture. This provided an opening to draw on constructs such as the culture-bound syndrome (CBS) and psychiatrist Peter D. Kramer's 'cosmetic psychopharmacology'.[1] In so doing, the interaction between norms of femininity and the diagnosis 'SAD' is investigated.

K. Masters, *Feminist and Anti-Psychiatry Perspectives on 'Social Anxiety Disorder'*,
https://doi.org/10.1007/978-3-031-48707-1_4

Diagnosis

The women I interviewed were a mixture of diagnosed and self-diagnosed, both with SAD and other psychiatric diagnoses. Amy spoke to my decision to include the testimonies of the self-diagnosed in this book after she highlighted the importance of her own diagnosis:

> [T]his is not to undercut anyone who identifies—mental health that hasn't been officially diagnosed—because obviously that gets into the difficulty of accessing healthcare, which is a whole other issue [...] So those people are obviously valid as well.

While accessing healthcare is a salient issue for all diagnoses, it is particularly impactful in terms of certain diagnoses. One such example, and one which is relevant for participant Phoebe, is Autism Spectrum Disorder (ASD). Unlike diagnoses which can be given and subsequently treated by a GP—like Generalised Anxiety Disorder[2] and Depression[3]—ASD can only be diagnosed by a specialist,[4] to whom one would need to be referred. Like talking therapies, waiting times for this are usually long[5] and provision is contingent on area.[6] As discussed earlier, all of these barriers to diagnosis have been buttressed by the Covid-19 pandemic. But there are yet more barriers for *women* in the case of ASD, for diagnosis is often not made in childhood: recent years have seen a growing number of women diagnosed later in life.[7] This trend rings true for Phoebe who, in her mid-twenties at interview, told me that she had 'never been diagnosed' with autism. Despite this, she predicted that a diagnosis would benefit her:

> I've been reading up a lot about it recently and I actually think that I am, it just makes so much sense to me [...] I'm thinking about going to try and get a diagnosis, just because it would [make] things feel like they fit in more, in my mind.

I mentioned in the previous chapter that, like Phoebe, I also suspect that I am autistic. For my part, when I dove deeper into descriptions of autism, the collection of disparate oddities I had always experienced began to make sense. To name but a few: seeing numbers and letters as particular colours,[8] being sensitive to noise, enjoying repeating certain words and phrases out loud, and cutting the last vestiges of labels out of all of my clothes lest I be unable to concentrate on anything other than the relentless scratchiness at the back of my neck. Rather than being peculiar to me, it seemed that these quirks were subsumed under an umbrella term and were common to other people—people like me.

As Phoebe imagined how a diagnosis would be beneficial, Amy spoke in similar terms about how her diagnoses of Depression and Anxiety actually *had* benefitted her:

> [H]aving that diagnosis changed a lot for me, because it allowed me to acknowledge it as a separate part of me and not just this weird, ambiguous, 'Why do I feel like this today?' [...] and that gives me something to hang onto [...] and a thing to look up.

Amy's and Phoebe's views on the utility of diagnosis mirror what clinical social worker Susan H. Berg describes as the typical liberal feminist position on PTSD. Berg contends that this position views diagnosis as useful to women insofar as it facilitates the development of treatment which helps them to 'continue to develop resources, both internal and external, to aid in their growth and fulfilment'.[9] By extension, diagnosis vis-à-vis mental distress more generally could be said to have utility because it identifies, names, and explains a particular type of experience.

As such, psychiatric diagnoses need not only pathologise and medicalise different ways of being—though do this they might—but can make possible 'the formation of a "reverse" discourse'.[10] Historian Rebecca Jennings draws on this Foucauldian idea in discussing female homosexuals who, in the nineteenth century, were termed 'inverts'.[11] Jennings challenges '[t]he idea that sexological categories were imposed on unwilling women by the hostile body of "experts"'.[12] She evidences this by citing several letters to the sexologist Edward Carpenter which 'suggest that individual women found the ideas of some sexologists helpful in thinking about their sexuality, but often as part of an ongoing process which had started prior to reading the literature'.[13] One woman 'described reading Carpenter's *The Intermediate Sex* as "like being given sight"';[14] another expressed that reading the opus 'had made her realise "that I myself belong to that class and [it] made everything fall into place"'.[15] This echoes Phoebe's sentiment that an ASD diagnosis would make things feel like they 'fit in more' for her. As such, while psychiatric diagnoses could be described as medicalising non-normativity, or as intelligible responses to gender-based trauma, they might equally be helpful in 'providing a name and framework'[16] for self-understanding—or, in Amy's words, they might give us 'something to hang on to'.

By contrast, Farah's perspective on being diagnosed with Anxiety is perhaps more reflective of Berg's description of the radical feminist position on the PTSD diagnosis, which views the label as pathologising. Farah explained:

> [T]hat kind of categorisation […] When they pathologise you, it actually increase[s] maybe, that anxiety […] Because you feel that, ok, you have [a] problem […] And thinking about solving that problem […] [i]ncrease[d] my anxiety.

Berg tells us that radical feminism holds that diagnosis and treatment pathologise women insofar as they 'ad[d] to the victim's belief in her defectiveness'.[17] As Farah related:

> Farah: [T]he doctor told me, 'Oh, why did you suffer this much? You could come sooner and we could solve it for you. By just using this medicine, 70% of this problem would be solved,' […] Lack of some—some er … Stuff in your body […]
>
> Katie: Oh, serotonin in your brain?
>
> Farah: Yeah, you know, and then, it's not all about your characteristic[s] or […] personality […] You would think that, ok, there's something different … There's something wrong with your body as well.

The prospect of being pathologised and, as Farah described, the resulting *increase* in anxiety, might offer yet *another* reason as to why participants typically did not seek help expressly for their social anxiety. The possibility of pathologisation might also be a deterrent for help-seeking if these women deemed their social anxiety to be another facet of their personality—as Farah and Ellen expressed—as opposed to an illness in need of treatment.[18] On treatment for SAD, there is a mode which surfaced in numerous participants' narratives and one which we have yet to discuss: talking therapies.

Therapy

Of the seven women I interviewed, Ria, Olivia, Daniella, and Amy had all engaged in talking therapy for their mental distress. For Amy, this was during her time spent living in the US and was with an art therapist, while the other three engaged in talking therapies while living in the UK. That only three of these women, of the five who had lived in the UK for their entire lives,[19] had received therapy while living in the UK speaks to points I made earlier: that therapy provision in the UK is patchy[20] and waiting lists are lengthy[21]—even more so in the wake of the Covid-19 pandemic. By contrast, five of the women I interviewed—Farah, Ellen, Olivia, Ria, and Daniella—had taken medication for their mental distress.[22] This reminds us of another point raised earlier: faced with long waiting lists and no alternative, GPs are prescribing more and more antidepressants.[23] This is perhaps a shame, since some of the women who had engaged with therapy described how it had helped them. Olivia shared her experience: 'The counselling helped with dealing with depression a little. I didn't do many sessions but the ones I did, I felt were helpful in just talking to someone about how I felt and being reminded of little self-care techniques.'

Amy's experience with an art therapist while living in the US was similar:

> I had a really good therapist for a couple of years there who gave me a lot of good resources [...] even just the awareness of like diagnostics [...] knowing what it is that makes your brain do what it does is a helpful tool to go, 'Oh, that's not really just me losing my mind, that's what Anxiety looks like.' Now let's acknowledge it [and] take steps to see what you can do to curb it.

With that said, therapy has been subject to critique in some feminist circles. That is not to suggest that these women are wrong for engaging in it or for finding it helpful: if it aids in alleviating distress, then its use should of course be applauded. Rather, some feminists have contended that therapy colludes with the psy sciences insofar as it 'provides individual approaches to collective problems ... [so that] each woman comes to see her problems as unique'.[24]

In the UK, guidelines for doctors recommend a type of therapy called cognitive behavioural therapy (CBT) for diagnoses germane to participants' experiences: SAD,[25] Depression,[26] Generalised Anxiety Disorder,[27] Anorexia Nervosa,[28] Bulimia Nervosa,[29] and Binge Eating Disorder.[30] Psychologist Ricki E. Kantrowitz and feminist therapist Mary Ballou, in their feminist critique of CBT, provide relevant commentary on this in arguing that therapy places the onus to adapt to the environment squarely on the shoulders of the individual.[31] Hence, 'the dominant social standards' remain unchallenged and are reinforced.[32] The assumption that it is they who needed to adapt was latent when Olivia and Amy spoke about therapy: both cited therapy as having given them tools with which to help themselves, but neither expressed that their therapy had addressed environmental issues. This surprised me somewhat: at other points in their interviews, both women described how their gendered socialisation had contributed to their social anxiety.

The question then remains: can the benefits of therapy be obtained while addressing external factors? Kantrowitz and Ballou argue that they can, if CBT were to be made more feminist. This would comprise examining the contexts of women's lives—'society, culture, [...] race, developmental status, and individual experiences'[33]—and environmental factors such as 'social and economic class, gender, ethnicity, political structures, and religion'.[34] In sum, CBT must 'attend to and develop programs aimed at altering the natural setting instead of changing the individual'.[35]

Kantrowitz and Ballou were writing their critique of CBT in 1992; Amy's and Olivia's descriptions of therapy, obtained from their interviews in 2018–2019, would support the view that it perhaps still has a way to go in terms of addressing the natural settings of women's lives. Until such a time that CBT achieves this, it is worth considering the viability of methods outside of the psy sciences. One example is talking with other socially anxious women. Recall that Olivia, in discussing the positive effects of counselling, stated that 'just talking to someone about how I felt' was beneficial. Likewise, Ria, who shared that she had 'had counselling', but had little to say on its specific effects, expressed an opinion similar to Olivia's:

> Ria: [I]t's kind of hard to apply logic to yourself [...] unless you write things down, to spot patterns. But when you talk to someone else [...] you can spot patterns in the outward behaviour [...]
>
> Katie: You mean like in terms of therapy?
>
> Ria: I think just generally, just generally conversing with someone you can pick things up [...] with yourself, you've kind of got your whole id and your inner world to contend with as well.

The therapeutic benefit garnered from speaking with someone trusted could therefore prove valuable for socially anxious women. This might be cathartic, as in the case of Olivia, or aid in spotting unhelpful patterns of thinking, as in the case of Ria. More broadly, simply conversing with someone who has experiences akin to one's own could mitigate sentiments which feed social anxiety: loneliness, being an outsider, or being different. The solidarity that talking with others confers could also remind socially anxious women that they are not at fault, and that their problems are not as individual as psy science conceptions would often have them believe.

While Olivia, Amy, and Ria had engaged with one of the two strands of SAD treatment in the UK (therapy),[36] Olivia, Ria, Daniella, Ellen, and Farah had engaged with the other: medication. Having discussed participants' views on therapy and, earlier, the backdrop against which antidepressants are prescribed—the biomedical model endorsed by psychiatry and big pharma—what remains is to engage with participants' perspectives on, and experiences with, these drugs.

Medication and Femininity

In discussing medication, it is necessary to home in on the neurotransmitter serotonin. This is often cited as culpable in mental distress and it is the basis on which many antidepressants are purported to work. By contrast, Irving Kirsch suggests that antidepressants, which usually act by increasing serotonin levels, are no more effective than placebo.[37] He also contends that their efficacy seems to be independent of whether they function to increase or decrease serotonin or act on a completely different neurotransmitter.[38] Studies have since tried to debunk Kirsch's claims,[39] but Kirsch, in response, maintains that 'most (if not all) of the benefits of antidepressants in the treatment of depression and anxiety are due to the placebo response'. That is, drugs' side effects mean that patients, and clinicians, can deduce who has been given the real drug and hence they 'break blind'.[40]

The account that Daniella initially gave of her antidepressant use was in alignment with the thoughts of Kirsch, for she told me, 'I started getting help from the GP and they put me on—they made me try medication, which, a year or so later, still doesn't really [laughs] [is] still not having a massive effect.' But Daniella's experience was layered: as we will see, she later talks of how she feels that antidepressants *have* helped her. This element was also to be found in Farah's testimony, since she was unsure whether she could attribute improvements to Zoloft:[41]

> Katie: [T]he medication, did you think it helped?
>
> Farah: I really don't know because [...] at the same time, lots of things changed in my life [...] at the same time I started to go to [the] gym.

And Ria's experience with antidepressants was mixed:

> I went on citalopram, briefly […] it didn't jive with me that well […] then went on fluoxetine. Jived a little better, found it was taking me a bit … Manic […] But I was better […] and it got to the point where […] I felt convicted of the decision to not take the tablets any further, so I just didn't—but it worked […] And the Bulimia sort of sorted itself out.

Olivia's account was also ambivalent, but in a different way. She shared her experience with the antidepressant sertraline: 'The medication has had a much more noticeable effect in helping my depression than in helping my social anxiety.' Although she did not elaborate as to why she thought this had been her experience, I cannot help but wonder whether the very name of this class of drugs—*antidepress*ants—might be thought to reflect their mechanism of action and hence their effects. Even if this association is unconscious, it might, following Kirsch, have helped to leverage the placebo effect in relieving some of Olivia's symptoms of depression, but not of her social anxiety.

Moving away from Kirch's tenets on the placebo effect, I wish to remind the reader of James Warner's observation vis-à-vis antidepressants: 'Looking at mean responses irons out those that don't respond at all and those that respond quite well.'[42] This is in line with Kramer's observations, since he characterises a number of the individuals he treated with antidepressants as 'good responders'.[43] On this point, Ellen spoke about how she has found the antidepressant fluoxetine to be very helpful:

> I found one that I like […] if I'm ok, I'll forget to take it and then I'll go like shit again, then I'm like 'Why am I shit?' and I'm like, 'Oh, it's because I've been okay, so I forgot to take the tablets.'

Despite the conflict in a number of these women's accounts, that several of them seem to have found antidepressants helpful problematises the idea that these medications are inherently anti-feminist or that they are opposed to anti-psychiatry-inspired conceptions of mental distress. What *is* objectionable is the viewpoint—arguably espoused by biological psychiatry and big pharma—that mental distress is solely biologically based and that antidepressants are a panacea for social problems, including mental distress arising from gender-based oppression.

Ellen spoke to these dominant narratives on antidepressants when she explained to me how she rationalised taking fluoxetine. Evoking the idea that 'mental illness' is an illness 'like any other',[44] she told me how she sometimes found herself thinking, 'I don't want to be reliant on these.' She then thought this through as follows: 'But then I'm like, "Ah, well if I was in pain I'd just be taking paracetamol." There's no difference.' Despite seeming to endorse the idea that mental distress is akin to physical pain, Ellen then pushed back against biological reductionism by acknowledging the social component of her mental distress, telling me, '[M]y insecurities are the result of what is going on in the world. Therefore, is it biological? No. I wouldn't feel this way if this wasn't happening.'

Framing 'mental illness' as an illness 'like any other'[45] is in keeping with the 'low serotonin' or 'chemical imbalance' model. A number of interviewees had something to say about this, not least Amy, whose faith in this model was evidenced by our exchange:

> Katie: [P]eople talk about mental health issues as a chemical imbalance in the brain or, kind of, low serotonin. I wondered what your take on that was, what you thought about that?
>
> Amy: I mean, I agree with science, if that's what you're asking [...] Yeah, definitely.

Amy's conviction in this model, on account of its being 'science', speaks to the Foucauldian idea that science has replaced religiosity as a tool of population control.[46] Besides this, Amy explained *why* she finds this model helpful:

> [T]he chemicals in the brain are what make me feel things and when they get out of whack, that's how depression and anxiety happen. That goes back to that burden of responsibility and that sort of shame that comes from, you know, 'I shouldn't feel sad, so why do I feel sad? I shouldn't feel anxious, so argh, why is this happening? [...]' And then I get mad at myself for feeling 'wrong'. So removing that burden of responsibility is a really important element, and chemical imbalance in the brain is literally the answer to that, right?

For Amy, the chemical imbalance model provides a reason, which is out of her control, as to why she feels 'wrong', or, I suggest, perhaps why she is *made* to feel 'wrong' by society. In seeking to understand further why Amy might find the idea of a chemical imbalance model useful, we can look to Angela Thachuk's thoughts on the biomedical model of 'mental illness'. That is, this model displaces

> [S]tigmatizing attitudes [...] from the individual onto the symptoms or behavioral manifestations of the illness. In theory, the integrity of one's character remains intact. She is not so much a deviant as much as she is one who, involuntarily, exhibits and/or undergoes deviant behaviors.[47]

Olivia's narrative also featured the chemical imbalance model, but she attributed her mental distress to it only in part, telling me, 'I'm still unsure if the depression is caused by chemical imbalances in the brain or by contraception or by environmental factors, or a mix of these.' Her words however echoed Amy's description of feeling 'wrong' insofar as she told me that 'the medication worked quickly in helping me feel more "normal" again, which really made me think my depression must be caused by a chemical imbalance in the brain'.

Both of these women mention there being a 'wrong' or 'normal' way of feeling. Here we have the idea that one must feel a certain way—'happy'—lest they are abnormal which, following Michel Foucault, is then conflated with being mentally 'sick'.[48] Simon J. Williams discusses the conflation of happiness with emotional health in arguing that

> [F]ar from being 'unhealthy' or 'pathological', it is indeed quite normal if not healthy to feel dissatisfied, disillusioned or even downright depressed at times; not simply due to prevailing ideologies of happiness and personal fulfilment, but also because of the embodied dilemmas and existential predicaments we all, qua human beings, inevitably face. We must not, in other words, confuse or equate issues of emotional health with happiness and wellbeing. Emotional health, in this sense, may indeed run the gamut of emotions, including those currently deemed 'treatable' by whatever means.[49]

If we are to apply Williams's tenets to Olivia's narrative, then her return to feeling 'normal', facilitated by medication, might not actually represent a return to emotional health. Rather, it could represent a return to what society sanctions as an appropriate emotional state: happiness or wellbeing.

I discussed earlier the work of psychiatrist Kramer in exploring how definitions of psychiatric disorders rest upon cultural norms.[50] Indeed, some people 'require' psychiatric treatment only because of a mismatch between their environment and their temperament.[51] Do Amy and Olivia therefore feel 'wrong', not how they 'should', or not 'normal' because society values certain traits in women? The current normative white femininity[52]—besides comprising 'youth, whiteness, slenderness, affluence, [and] able-bodiedness'—consists of 'erotic interest in men' and, crucially, '*extroversion*'.[53] The latter two traits are especially unlikely to be patent in the socially anxious, or depressed, woman.

Viewing Amy's embracing of the chemical imbalance model in light of these feminine norms, it becomes clear why this explanation might be helpful to avoid self-blame. If her personality style and feminine ideals—particularly the currently *en vogue* 'masculine femininity', as previously defined—do not match up, the chemical imbalance model provides a means by which she can navigate this discord without subscribing to the idea that her temperament is at fault.

Olivia's statement that taking antidepressants made her feel 'normal' again has further relevance to the thoughts of Kramer, for he contends that an antidepressant has the potential to alter personality style. In so doing, this prescription could be viewed as bringing the individual in line with the current feminine ideal—comprising 'behaviour and decorum in service of white masculinity'[54]—and thereby endorsing 'a certain sort of social conformity'.[55] If there is no longer conflict between how a woman feels and how she is persistently told by society that she *ought* to feel, she might well feel 'normal' again, as Olivia described.

Although Daniella did not speak explicitly about feeling 'wrong', or the chemical imbalance model, her antidepressant use bears resemblance to that of Olivia. Daniella spoke about her experience *prior* to taking medication:

> I used to be really obsessed about what people thought of me [...] if I was in an awkward situation, I would feel like I was cringing inside [...] I would get really anxious [...] I would feel really bad if I made a mistake, or if I had to explain myself [...] Dwell on it massively, I could not have a conversation without like [...] crying [...] I used to care far too much about absolutely everything.

Some of the personality traits which Daniella is describing evoke what Kramer describes as 'Victorian femininity', elements of which include being 'emotionally sensitive', 'fastidious', and 'melancholic'.[56] Her description also calls to mind several of the feminine attributes within Sandra L. Bem's Sex Role Inventory: being shy, soft spoken, yielding, eager to soothe hurt feelings, and sensitive to the needs of others.[57]

Daniella then described the changes that medication has made: '[T]he abrupt mood changes have gone [...] It's more stable in the sense that I don't like cry for no reason all the time [...] I don't care as much.' Now, Daniella's personality style features what Kramer describes as traditionally 'masculine' traits,[58] or the masculine elements in what I have termed 'masculine femininity'. These characteristics include 'resilience, energy, assertiveness, an enjoyment of give-and-take';[59] being vivacious and mentally quick;[60] and being analytical.[61] Her temperament is now also reminiscent of sociologist Anita Harris's exposition of modern young adult femininity in the early twenty-first century, which can be found in the 'can-do' girl. This type of girl is characterised by confidence and resilience[62] and has much in common with the 'the ideal late[-]modern subject [...] who is flexible, individualized, resilient, self-driven, and self-made and who easily follows nonlinear trajectories to fulfillment and success'.[63] The 'can-do' girls, therefore,

> [A]re identifiable by their commitment to exceptional careers and career planning, their belief in their capacity to invent themselves and succeed, and their display of a consumer lifestyle. They are also distinguished by a desire to put off childbearing until 'later'. [...] This is a sexy, brash, and individualized expression of ambition, power, and success [...] drawn from a wide range of areas: girls' educational success; their consumption, leisure, and fashion practices; apparent rejection of institutionalized feminism; sexual assertiveness; professional ambitions; delayed motherhood, and so on.[64]

The construction of this kind of femininity, Harris argues, creates 'docile good girls who can uncomplainingly participate in meeting the needs of the marketplace'.[65] This resonates with Daniella's experience of some of the changes she felt on taking medication, which she described as having 'helped for some things. I'm definitely able to do some work [...] whereas before, I just could not'. Daniella continued with this thread in describing an instance when she was reprimanded at work and how this did not bother her. She followed this by telling me how this would have played out had it occurred prior to her taking medication:

> I would have cried on the spot for ages and I would've felt like crap for [...] the rest of the day [...] it would have been, 'Oh, I'm a failure. That's it. There's nothing you can do about it: you suck.'

This aspect of Daniella's testimony calls to mind Kramer's question as to whether medicating women with antidepressants enforces adherence to '"masculine" capitalist values' in order to serve society's economic needs.[66] Indeed, Farah spoke to this more explicitly in explaining to me that, in the context of her home country in Western Asia, shyness is 'consider[ed] as a kind of virtue' and is '[p]raised, for women. As a kind of "good woman", kind of "moral"'. Crucially, she added that 'now, I think they are moving from that stage, because women are also supposed to be successful in this capitalistic system. So, they don't have this chance of even being shy'.

In considering capitalism and the workplace, Harris's citing of cultural and feminist theorist Angela McRobbie becomes relevant. That is, '[I]mproving oneself is necessary to success in the labor and consumer markets'[67] for young women. Self-improvement was evident in Daniella's narrative, wherein she elaborated on being reproached at work: '[I]t's something that I need to change and I have to work on [...] I'm going to take action of this meeting, work on it, do whatever they say that I have to do.'

Another domain where the 'can-do' feminine ideal functions to meet the demands of the labour market is in the pressure to put off childbearing. This has required 'a reshaping of traditional conservative family values around mothering to accommodate the neoliberal agenda that calls for young women to function as high-status workers'.[68] However, women must 'delay childbearing until their careers are established but not [...] renounce motherhood altogether'.[69] The pressure to meet this requirement came through when I spoke to Farah, who was in her late thirties at interview:

> My mum, each time that she calls me, always tells me that, 'You should have children' [...] occasionally some friends [...] they would say, ok, because my husband also is younger than me [...] if one day he wants [children], then maybe he would leave you.

Harris tells us that women are 'simultaneously told that they must pursue careers and at the same time factor in children before it is "too late"'.[70] Lisa Downing has written on this 'double-bind', for she describes how '[t]he childless or childfree woman is othered as abnormal while the obediently reproductive woman, whose role is to provide infinite love, will be endlessly monitored, critiqued, and policed'.[71] She continues:

> [W]hile childfree women are routinely demonized for rejecting the role that has traditionally been seen as a woman's 'proper' one, women who do become mothers are not exempt from similar charges and also face grueling amounts of cultural surveillance regarding their level of commitment to motherhood, measured by the various associations that accrue to staying at home or working outside of the home in the popular cultural and media contexts and, in psychiatric and psychological ones, by suspicions of narcissistic mothering and 'helicopter parenting'.[72]

The contradictory expectations about which Harris and Downing write are at the very heart of feminine ideals at the time of writing this book. Women must exhibit 'desirable' masculine traits, as exemplified by 'masculine femininity', while still being seen as feminine 'enough'. Worry about leaning too far in either direction is quite understandable, as is worry about the negative evaluation that will ensue *no matter what a woman does*.

The impossible task of trying to strike this delicate balance calls to mind a tension of yesteryear: the conflict between Victorian femininity and the femininity of the 'New Woman' of the *fin de siècle*. In contrast with Victorian femininity, the New Woman had feminist politics; was independent, career-minded, and educated;[73] and her riding of bicycles was reflective of both her contravention of a woman's traditional gender role and her ability to engage with the world beyond the domestic sphere.[74] Incidentally, the New Woman was associated with nervous illness.[75] The conflict between these femininities evokes a tension which finds a place in the twentieth century. As psychiatrist P. Susan Penfold and social work scholar Gillian Walker note, women participating in consciousness-raising groups would often feel 'torn between a pull to remain with traditional ties and a pull to move onward'.[76] For Olivia, this tension has made it through to the twenty-first century:

> [G]rowing up I received confusing mixed messages about gender roles. It was seen as 'normal' and 'natural' in media, culture and everyday life that as a girl I would show attributes of being quiet, self-conscious, sensitive, thoughtful, sweet and caring, rather than confident, independent and assertive. Yet, at the same time there was the 'girls can do anything' narrative—messages that I think only superficially attempted to empower girls, because the traditional feminine roles of passivity and beauty were and are still very much alive. I think these messages about your prescribed gender role are overwhelming and make you set ridiculously high standards for yourself which are unattainable and that makes you feel personally inadequate.

The shallow rhetoric to which Olivia refers is visible in media in campaigns such as Sport England's *This Girl Can*[77] and Caryl Hart's book *Girls Can Do Anything!*[78] Although these examples are well-meaning, their message does not match up with most women's socialisation. There is, in the words of gender and media scholar Shani Orgad, 'a contradiction between representation and experience'.[79] While women are socialised to behave in one way, contrasting traits are held up as something towards which we should aspire. This is surely a recipe for women's not feeling good enough and, in turn, likely creates concern about what others might think.

The expectation that women exhibit contrasting—that is, masculine and feminine—characteristics is especially prominent in the workplace. Derald Wing Sue explains how

> These double standards create no-win situations for women. While men are valued for their assertiveness, an attribute of leadership, women evidencing these traits are described as 'bitchy'. Ironically, women are also aware that they must conform to masculine roles or behavior standards in order to be perceived as credible leaders. They are told to be wary of showing emotions or social sensitivities to others or they will be perceived as being 'weak' or 'too emotional' to deal with the rough and tumble of logical decisions.[80]

I am reminded here of Phylis Chesler's exposition of psychologist Inge K. Broverman et al.'s study,[81] wherein physicians' definitions of the 'healthy man' and 'healthy adult' were found to be one and the same. These stood in contradistinction to their definition of 'healthy woman', which was more emotional, dependent, and deferential while being less objective. Sue mentions this very same study in exploring femininity in the workplace:

> If 'male characteristics' denote health and effectiveness in the workforce, it means that 'healthy female traits' connote dysfunction and ineffectiveness in work situations. However, if women exhibit assertiveness at a work site (healthy male and healthy adult traits) she runs the risk of being perceived as an unhealthy female ('bitchy' or being 'butch').[82]

Business executive Sheryl Sandberg also writes on this phenomenon in pointing out 'the unfairness of women leaders being perceived as "unlikeable,"[83] while "men are continually applauded for being ambitious and powerful"'.[84] Moreover, as Downing notes, '"[N]ot being nice" is a feature of being human for which women are particularly harshly punished.'[85] As such, this 'no-win' situation, and the resulting spectre of not being liked, might stoke up fear regarding self-portrayal, and hence social anxiety, for women. Indeed, this was something to which Phoebe alluded when I asked her, '[W]hat do you think makes women vulnerable to social anxiety, especially?' She replied: 'I think … Especially is that women kind of can't win.'

Olivia's testimony more overtly connected these conflicting discourses on femininity with social anxiety: recall that she told me how 'these messages about your prescribed gender role are overwhelming and make you set ridiculously high standards for yourself which are unattainable and that makes you feel personally inadequate'. These feelings of inadequacy, which are born of women's socialisation and are so very intrinsic to social anxiety, were patent in many of the women's narratives in the preceding chapter. But these feelings can be explored further through the lens of Harris's 'can-do' femininity, since this brand of femininity holds that success is 'achieved through personal effort alone'[86] and 'good personal choices'.[87] Conversely, failure results from 'individual weakness',[88] for problems are viewed as personal in both 'cause and solution'.[89] In much the same way that the psy sciences endorse the individual pathology model in addressing mental distress, 'can-do' femininity posits that any (perceived) shortcomings are individual deficits: socialisation or structural inequalities are not factored into the analysis. Ria articulated the effects of these discourses in discussing her perception that she ought to be good at public speaking:

> [I]f I know I'm not good at something, I have to try and be better […] that kind of feeds it because I suppose you're more likely to put yourself in situations, perversely, that might stoke up a bit of social anxiety.

Olivia's and Ria's narratives not only communicate feelings of inadequacy but also betray discomfort about having weaknesses. This mirrors Harris's observation that the literature for and about girls is 'chock-full of workbook things you can do to improve yourself',[90] with magazines targeted at teenage girls starting 'from the supposition that girls need fixing'.[91] And whereas the pressures on girls prior to the advent of 'can-do' femininity might have said 'you're not thin enough or pretty enough',[92] they now seem to be saying, '[Y]ou're not strong enough or confident enough.'[93] Hence, the particular set of characteristics which women, even younger women, are expected to exhibit is no longer limited to physicality but incorporates the girl in her entirety. The result, as is evident in Ria's and Olivia's accounts, is 'the never-good-enough girl who must perpetually observe and remake herself'[94]—a never-ending project pursued in order to stave off apprehension about others' perceptions.

Since ideals of femininity now extend beyond physicality, one of the areas subsumed under their remit is academic success. For young women, this has 'become the key to safeguarding the future'.[95] Not only is it regarded as beneficial for the woman herself insofar as it facilitates her obtaining 'an appropriate adult professional and consumer life-style',[96] it supposedly prevents 'disaffection, criminality, and disenfranchisement'.[97] Along with the more traditional requirement that women emulate beauty ideals, Farah's narrative highlighted the importance placed on academic performance when she remembered how others evaluated her as a child: 'I didn't consider as an important kid in that family. Not beautiful, not important, and that beauty and smartness was important in that family.'

'Can-do' femininity holds that failure to reach these ideals—which run the gamut from beauty to smartness—results from individual failings and lack of 'good personal choices'.[98] The self is therefore presented as a project on which one should work.[99] Likewise, social historian Joan Jacobs Brumberg has termed girls' attempts at *physical* self-improvement 'the body project'.[100] It would be remiss not to mention cosmetic surgery at this juncture, and this evokes what Kramer has conceptualised as its parallel: '[C]osmetic psychopharmacology'[101]—the 'reshaping of personality traits by medication'.[102] This provides a convenient segue not only into reprising my discussion of prescribed psychiatric drugs, but also into discussing *non*-prescribed drugs as they pertain to participants' experiences.

Drugs

Earlier on, I relayed Olivia's experience of the antidepressant sertraline: '[T]he medication worked quickly in helping me feel more "normal" again.' Kramer notes that, likewise, people's motivation for taking *non*-prescribed drugs is oftentimes to 'feel normal'.[103] As such, Kramer questions whether street drugs and antidepressants are not 'morally indistinguishable in terms of the reasons they are taken and the results they produce'.[104] He asks 'whether street-drug abusers are self-medicating'[105] their mental distress and 'whether prescribed-drug users are, with their doctors' permission, stimulating and calming themselves in quite similar ways'.[106] Prescribed drug use could then be described as 'drug abuse' having 'sneaked through the back door',[107] since 'entering the middle class carries the privilege of access to socially sanctioned drugs that are safer and more specific in their effects than street drugs'.[108]

Since we are discussing drug use, it is worth touching upon the *DSM-5*'s position that 'Substance Abuse' is often 'co-morbid' with SAD.[109] However, only Farah mentioned having used a non-prescribed substance recreationally,[110] telling me:

> Farah: I was so comfortable with using drugs as well when I was young to help myself [...] For a short time, for example, I used opium, and opium is, you know, nice.
>
> Katie: Oh, really? Okay ... Did it help?
>
> Farah: Very much so! [laughs] [...] other drugs [weren't] helpful [...] grass or these kind of ... Weed [...] they are mostly considered as a kind of ... 'Hyper' drug, it makes you hyper ... So this is not good for me [...] I need something like opium, that category, that makes me ... Calm and opium is the best one ... And, of course, whenever I've used, I've done it among my friends so it's a very nice environment.

As opposed to fitting the *DSM-5*'s narrative on substance use and social anxiety, namely that '[s]elf-medication with substances is common (e.g., drinking before going to a party)',[111] Farah's account of opium use among friends seems akin to normative alcohol use at parties.

On alcohol, Farah also had an interesting perspective insofar as it allayed her social anxiety, for she told me, 'I'm much [more] comfortable in speaking when I'm drunk.' Interestingly, it was not the *direct* effect of alcohol which alleviated her social anxiety, as she explained:

> [W]hen people think that you are drunk, sometimes I even pretend that I am drunk, more than what I am, because people's expectations become lower [...] and you are more comfortable to [...] [say] what you want to say. You have more freedom if people think that you are drunk.

There are echoes here of my earlier discussion of Selective Mutism, in which Farah's narrative also featured. Recall that others' expectations that people with SM will not speak buttressed the barriers to speaking that they experienced. In much the same way, others' evaluations of Farah become altered when they believe her to be intoxicated. Therefore, if their evaluations are negative, as the socially anxious fear, then the intoxication offers a way out. The negative evaluation is not a reflection of a 'defect' in her personality, but is attributable to her inebriation. As individuals with SM feel shackled by others' expectations of them, Farah is describing alcohol use as a means by which she can free herself from the restrictions on her behaviours that others' expectations present.

As Substance Abuse is reported by the *DSM-5* as being 'co-morbid' with SAD, there is another diagnosis which falls into this category which I have yet to explore: Body Dysmorphic Disorder (BDD).[112] Ellen very briefly alluded to BDD by name in describing self-consciousness about her body—'[I] n my head I'm like, "Why do I even have that like—almost body dysmorphia?"'—though did not explicitly express that she identified with the diagnosis. Despite this, Farah, Daniella, Ellen, Phoebe, Olivia, and Ria, to varying degrees, all mentioned concern with how they look during their interviews; Daniella, Phoebe, and Ria also gave poignant accounts of their struggles with eating which were inextricable from their body image concerns. The next chapter will delve into how these appearance-centric types of mental distress relate to social anxiety.

Notes

1. Peter D. Kramer, *Listening to Prozac* (London: Fourth Estate, 1994), p. xvi.
2. NHS, *Do I Have an Anxiety Disorder?* (2018) https://www.nhs.uk/common-health-questions/lifestyle/do-i-have-an-anxiety-disorder/ [accessed 7 January 2021].
3. NHS, *Diagnosis: Clinical Depression* (2019) https://www.nhs.uk/conditions/clinical-depression/diagnosis/ [accessed 7 January 2021].
4. NHS, *How To Get Diagnosed* (2019) https://www.nhs.uk/conditions/autism/getting-diagnosed/how-to-get-diagnosed/ [accessed 25 September 2020].
5. Ibid.
6. National Autistic Society, *Pre-diagnosis Support – A Guide for Adults Who Think They Might Be Autistic* (2020) https://www.autism.org.uk/about/diagnosis/adults.aspx [accessed 25 September 2020].
7. Sarah Bargiela, Robyn Steward, and William Mandy, 'The Experiences of Late-diagnosed Women with Autism Spectrum Conditions: An Investigation of the Female Autism Phenotype', *Journal of Autism and Developmental Disorders*, 46.10 (2016), 3281–94 https://doi.org/10.1007/s10803-016-2872-8
For more on the sociological and cultural factors shaping women's lower rates of ASD diagnosis, see Liane Holliday Willey, *Pretending To Be Normal: Living with Asperger's Syndrome* (London/Philadelphia: Jessica

Kingsley Publishers, 2015) and Rudy Simone, *Aspergirls* (London/ Philadelphia: Jessica Kingsley Publishers, 2010).

8. This is called 'synaesthesia'. Although it is not a 'symptom' of autism, it has been found to be relatively common in autistic individuals. See Olga Bogdashina, 'Synaesthesia in Autism', *National Autistic Society* (2016) https://www.autism.org.uk/advice-and-guidance/professional-practice/synaesthesia [accessed 21 June 2023].
9. Sandra Bloom, *Creating Sanctuary* (New York: Routledge, 1997).
   Judith Lewis Herman, 'Complex PTSD: A Syndrome in Survivors of Prolonged and Repeated Trauma', *Journal of Traumatic Stress*, 3 (1992), 377–91 https://doi.org/10.1002/jts.2490050305
   Irene P. Stiver, 'The Meaning of Care: Reframing Treatment Models', in *Women's Growth in Connection*, ed. by Irene P. Stiver, Judith V. Jordan, Jean Baker Miller, Janet Surrey, and Alexandra G. Kaplan (New York: Guilford, 1991), 250–67.
   Lenore E. Walker, *Abused Women and Survivor Therapy: A Practical Guide for the Psychotherapist* (Washington, DC: American Psychological Association, 1994).
   All cited in Susan H. Berg, 'The PTSD Diagnosis: Is It Good for Women?', *Affilia*, 17.1 (2002), 55–68 https://doi.org/10.1177/088610990201700l004 p. 58.
10. Michel Foucault, *The Will to Knowledge, The History of Sexuality: I*, trans. Robert Hurley (Harmondsworth: Penguin, 1998), p. 101.
11. Rebecca Jennings, *A Lesbian History of Britain: Love and Sex between Women Since 1500* (Oxford/Westport, Connecticut: Greenwood World Publishing, 2007), p. 77.
12. Ibid., pp. 86–87.
13. Ibid., p. 87.
14. George Meredith, *Diary of the Crossways* (London: Virago, 1980 [1885]), pp. 41, 132, cited in Sally Ledger, *The New Woman: Fiction and Feminism at the Fin de Siècle* (Manchester: Manchester University Press, 1991), p. 135, cited in Jennings, *A Lesbian History of Britain*, p. 88.
15. Liz Stanley, 'Romantic Friendship? Some Issues in Researching Lesbian History and Biography', *Women's History Review*, 1.2 (1992), 193–216 https://doi.org/10.1080/0961202920010201 pp. 206–08, cited in Jennings, *A Lesbian History of Britain*, pp. 87–88.
16. Edward Carpenter Archive Letters, 386.218, 386.262, 386.355, 386.409, cited in Jennings, *A Lesbian History of Britain*, p. 88.
17. Berg, 'The PTSD Diagnosis', p. 61.
18. For a more in-depth analysis of this issue, see Katie Masters, 'Women's Experiences of Social Anxiety Disorder: Privileging Marginalised Perspectives and Rewriting Dominant Narratives', *International Mad*

Studies Journal, 1.1 (2022), e1–21 https://doi.org/10.58544/imsj.v1i1.5244

19. In terms of participants who had moved to the UK from other countries, Daniella had lived in the UK for seven years and Farah had lived in the UK for at least three years at the time of interview.
20. Mind, *We Need To Talk: Getting the Right Therapy at the Right Time* (n.d.) https://www.mind.org.uk/media/280583/We-Need-to-Talk-getting-the-right-therapy-at-the-right-time.pdf [accessed 10 June 2019] p. 7.
    NHS England, *Adult Improving Access to Psychological Therapies Programme* (n.d.) https://www.england.nhs.uk/mental-health/adults/iapt/ [accessed 7 January 2021].
21. Julia Hyde, Michael Calnan, Lindsay Prior, Glyn Lewis, David Kessler, and Deborah Sharp, 'A Qualitative Study Exploring how GPs Decide To Prescribe Antidepressants', *British Journal of General Practice*, 55.519 (2005), 755–62 https://www.ncbi.nlm.nih.gov/pmc/articles/PMC1562347/ [accessed 25 September 2020] pp. 759–60.
    Royal Pharmaceutical Society, 'Most GPs are Over-prescribing Antidepressants', *The Pharmaceutical Journal Online*, 272.7293 (2004), 407 https://www.pharmaceutical-journal.com/pj-online-news-most-gps-are-over-prescribing-antidepressants/20011591.article?firstPass=false [accessed 10 June 2019].
    Emily Wooster on behalf of the We Need To Talk campaign, *While We are Waiting: Experiences of Waiting for and Receiving Psychological Therapies on the NHS* (2019) https://www.mentalhealth.org.uk/publications/while-we-are-waiting [accessed 10 June 2019] p. 8.
22. For Farah, this was both during her time living in Western Asia and the UK.
23. Ibid.
    Gareth Iacobucci, 'NHS Prescribed Record Number of Antidepressants Last Year', *British Medical Journal*, 364.1508 (2019) https://doi.org/10.1136/bmj.l1508
24. J. Arches, 'Women and Mental Health', *Catalyst: A Socialist Journal of the Social Services*, 4 (1984), 43–57, p. 49, cited in Janet A. Nes and Peter Iadicola, 'Toward a Definition of Feminist Social Work: A Comparison of Liberal, Radical, and Socialist Models', *Social Work*, 34.1 (1989), 12–21 http://www.jstor.org/stable/23715611 [accessed 19 June 2023].
25. NICE, *Interventions for Adults with Social Anxiety Disorder* (2013) https://www.nice.org.uk/guidance/cg159/chapter/1-Recommendations#interventions-for-adults-with-social-anxiety-disorder-2 [accessed 25 September 2020].
    N. B.: Short-term psychodynamic psychotherapy is also recommended for SAD specifically.

26. NICE, *Depression in Adults: Recognition and Management* (2009) https://www.nice.org.uk/guidance/cg90/chapter/1-Guidance#treatment-choice-based-on-depression-subtypes-and-personal-characteristics [accessed 25 September 2020].
27. NICE, *Principles of Care for People with Generalised Anxiety Disorder (GAD)* (2019) https://www.nice.org.uk/guidance/cg113/chapter/1-Guidance#principles-of-care-for-people-with-generalised-anxiety-disorder-gad [accessed 25 September 2020].
28. NICE, *Treating Anorexia Nervosa* (2020) https://www.nice.org.uk/guidance/ng69/chapter/Recommendations#treating-anorexia-nervosa [accessed 17 May 2023].
29. NICE, *Treating Bulimia Nervosa* (2020) https://www.nice.org.uk/guidance/ng69/chapter/Recommendations#treating-bulimia-nervosa [accessed 7 January 2021].
30. NICE, *Treating Binge Eating Disorder* (2020) https://www.nice.org.uk/guidance/ng69/chapter/Recommendations#treating-binge-eating-disorder [accessed 17 May 2023].
31. Ricki E. Kantrowitz and Mary Ballou, 'A Feminist Critique of Cognitive Behavioral Therapy', in *Personality and Psychopathology: Feminist Reappraisals*, ed. by Laura S Brown and Mary B. Ballou (New York: The Guilford Press, 1992), 70–87, pp. 77, 79, 83.
32. Ibid.
33. Ibid., p. 82.
34. Ibid., p. 84.
35. Ibid., p. 86.
36. NICE, *Interventions for Adults with Social Anxiety Disorder.*
37. Kirsch, 'Antidepressants and the Placebo Effect', *ZeitschriftfürPsychologie*, 222.3 (2014), 128–34 https://doi.org/10.1027/2151-2604/a000176 p. 128.
38. Ibid.
39. E.g. Andrea Cipriani, Toshi A. Furukawa, Georgia Salanti, Anna Chaimani, Lauren Z. Atkinson, Yusuke Ogawa, Stefan Leucht, Henricus G. Ruhe, Erick H. Turner, Julian P. T. Higgins, Matthias Egger, Nozomi Takeshima, Yu Hayasaka, Hissei Imai, Kiyomi Shinohara, Aran Tajika, John P. A. Ioannidis, and John R. Geddes, 'Comparative Efficacy and Acceptability of 21 Antidepressant Drugs for the Acute Treatment of Adults with Major Depressive Disorder: A Systematic Review and Network Meta-analysis', *Focus*, 16.4 (2018), 420–29 https://doi.org/10.1176/appi.focus.16407
40. Irving Kirsch, 'Placebo Effect in the Treatment of Depression and Anxiety', *Frontiers in Psychiatry*, 10.407 (2019) https://doi.org/10.3389/fpsyt.2019.00407

41. The generic name for which is 'sertraline', an SSRI.
42. Clare Wilson, 'Nobody Can Agree about Antidepressants'.
43. Kramer, *Listening to Prozac*, p. 236.
44. Hyman, quoted in Albee and Joffe, 'Mental illness Is NOT an "Illness Like Any Other"', cited in Brett J. Deacon, 'The Biomedical Model of Mental Disorder: A Critical Analysis of its Validity, Utility, and Effects on Psychotherapy Research', *Clinical Psychology Review*, 33.7 (2013), 846–61 https://doi.org/10.1016/j.cpr.2012.09.007 pp. 851–52.
45. Ibid.
46. Michel Foucault, *Ethics: Subjectivity and Truth: Essential Works of Michel Foucault 1954–1984, Vol. 1*, ed. by Paul Rabinow, trans. Robert Hurley and others (New York: The New Press, 1997), p. 313.
47. Angela K. Thachuk, 'Stigma and the Politics of Biomedical Models of Mental Illness', *International Journal of Feminist Approaches to Bioethics*, 4.1 (2011), 140–63 https://doi.org/10.3138/ijfab.4.1.140 p. 150.
48. Michel Foucault, 'Je Suis un Artificier', in *Michel Foucault, Entretiens*, ed. by Roger-Pol Droit (Paris: Odile Jacob, 2004), p. 95.
49. Simon J. Williams, 'Reason, Emotion and Embodiment: Is "Mental" Health a Contradiction in Terms?', *Sociology of Health and Illness*, 22.5 (2000), 559–81 https://doi.org/10.1111/1467-9566.00220 p. 572.
50. Kramer, *Listening to Prozac*, p. xv.
51. Ibid., p. 246.
52. Kathy Deliovsky, 'Normative White Femininity: Race, Gender and the Politics of Beauty', *Atlantis: Critical Studies in Gender, Culture and Social Justice*, 33.1 (2008), 49–59 https://journals.msvu.ca/index.php/atlantis/article/view/429 [accessed 30 January 2023].
53. Laura T. Hamilton, Elizabeth A. Armstrong, J. Lotus Seeley, and Elizabeth M. Armstrong, 'Hegemonic Femininities and Intersectional Domination', *Sociological Theory*, 37.4 (2019), 315–41 https://doi.org/10.1177/0735275119888248 p. 325. My emphasis.
54. Deliovsky, 'Normative White Femininity', p. 57.
55. Kramer, *Listening to Prozac*, p. 271.
56. Ibid.
57. Sandra L. Bem, 'The Measurement of Psychological Androgyny', *Journal of Consulting and Clinical Psychology*, 42.2 (1974), 155–62 https://doi.org/10.1037/h0036215 p. 156.
58. Kramer, *Listening to Prozac*, p. 271.
59. Ibid.
60. Ibid., p. 270.
61. Bem, 'The Measurement of Psychological Androgyny', p. 156.

62. Anita Harris, *Future Girl: Young Women in the Twenty-first Century* (Taylor and Francis Group, 2003) https://ebookcentral.proquest.com/lib/bham/reader.action?docID=182880 [accessed 25 September 2020] p. 13.
63. Ibid., p. 16.
64. Ibid., pp. 13–17.
65. Ibid., p. 18.
66. Kramer, *Listening to Prozac*, p. 271.
67. Harris, *Future Girl*, p. 19.
68. Ibid., p. 21.
69. Ibid., p. 21.
70. Ibid., p. 23.
71. Lisa Downing, *Selfish Women* (Abingdon, Oxon; New York, NY: Routledge, 2019), p. 101.
72. Ibid., p. 3.
73. Hugh Stevens, *Henry James and Sexuality* (Cambridge: Cambridge University Press, 2008), p. 27.
74. Jacob Roberts, 'Women's Work', *Distillations*, 3.1 (2017), 6–11 https://www.sciencehistory.org/distillations/womens-work [accessed 25 September 2020].
75. Elaine Showalter, *The Female Malady: Women, Madness, and English Culture* (New York: Pantheon, 1985), p. 137.
76. P. Susan Penfold and Gillian Walker, *Women and the Psychiatric Paradox* (Milton Keynes: Open University Press, 1984), p. 219.
77. Sport England, *This Girl Can* (n.d.) https://www.thisgirlcan.co.uk/ [accessed 25 September 2020].
78. Caryl Hart, *Girls Can Do Anything!* (Southam: Scholastic, 2018).
79. Shani Orgad, *Heading Home: Motherhood, Work, and the Failed Promise of Equality* (New York; Chichester, West Sussex: Columbia University Press, 2019), pp. 40–41.
80. Derald Wing Sue, *Microaggressions in Everyday Life: Race, Gender, and Sexual Orientation* (John Wiley and Sons Incorporated, 2010) https://ebookcentral.proquest.com/lib/bham/reader.action?docID=487711 [accessed 24 September 2020] p. 163.
81. Inge K. Broverman, Donald M. Broverman, Frank E. Clarkson, Paul S. Rosenkrantz, and Susan R. Vogel, 'Sex-role Stereotypes and Clinical Judgments of Mental Health', *Journal of Consulting and Clinical Psychology*, 34.1 (1970), 1–7 https://doi.org/10.1037/h0028797 cited in Phyllis Chesler, *Women and Madness* (London: Allen Lane, 1974), p. 65.
82. Sue, *Microaggressions*, pp. 165–66.
83. Sheryl Sandberg, *Lean In: Women, Work and the Will To Lead* (New York: WH Allen, 2013), loc. 2400, cited in Downing, *Selfish Women*, p. 119.

84. Sandberg, *Lean In*, loc. 253, cited in Downing, *Selfish Women*, p. 119.
85. Downing, *Selfish Women*, p. 152.
86. Harris, *Future Girl*, p. 19.
87. Ibid., p. 31.
88. Angela McRobbie, 'Good Girls, Bad Girls? Female Success and the New Meritocracy', unpublished keynote address presented at *A New Girl Order?* conference, London, 14–16 November 2001, cited in Harris, *Future Girl*, p. 19.
89. Harris, *Future Girl*, p. 33.
90. Ibid., p. 32.
91. Ibid.
92. Jennifer Baumgardner and Amy Richards, *Manifesta: Young Women, Feminism and the Future* (New York: Farrar, Straus and Giroux, 2001), p. 191.
93. Ibid.
94. Harris, *Future Girl*, p. 32.
95. Ibid., p. 27.
96. Ibid.
97. Ibid.
98. Ibid., p. 31.
99. Ibid., p. 32.
100. Joan Jacobs Brumberg, *The Body Project: An Intimate History of American Girls* (New York: Vintage Books, 1998).
101. Kramer, *Listening to Prozac*, p. xvi.
102. Ibid., p. 143.
103. Kramer, *Listening to Prozac*, p. 16.
104. Ibid.
105. Ibid.
106. Ibid.
107. Ibid.
108. Ibid.
109. American Psychiatric Association [APA], *Diagnostic and Statistical Manual of Mental Disorders* [*DSM-5*] (Washington, DC: American Psychiatric Association Publishing, 2013) https://ebookcentral.proquest.com/lib/bham/reader.action?docID=1811753 [accessed 6 January 2021] p. 208.
110. The illegality of substances in the UK at the time of writing, coupled with the lack of social acceptability of drug use—specifically in the case of women—may have precluded other participants from sharing their experiences in this regard.
111. Ibid., p. 204.
112. Ibid., p. 208.

CHAPTER 5

Watching Women's Bodies, Watching Women's Selves

For several of the women I interviewed, fear of negative evaluation was felt most deeply when it came to their appearance, their body, and their size—the first half of this chapter sees this interplay fleshed out. Despite the body seemingly being a mainstay of the socially anxious woman's experience, interviewees indicated that their apprehension about others' appraisals often extended to how they were perceived as a whole person. The chapter's second half therefore frames women's social anxiety as the fear of their *entire performance* being negatively evaluated. As participants expressed these ideas, social media was recurrently cited as compounding, and being intertwined with, their difficulties. It therefore forms a motif throughout this whole chapter.

Things of Beauty

The imperative to adhere to a physical ideal was a tie which bound many participants' experiences. Kathy Deliovsky has written on this ideal, noting 'the white capitalist patriarchal compulsion to adopt styles and attitudes consistent with an imposed white feminine aesthetic'.[1] Similarly, sociologist Raewyn Connell has termed the culturally valued form of femininity 'emphasized femininity', and argues that it is 'defined around compliance with subordination and is oriented to accommodating the interests and

K. Masters, *Feminist and Anti-Psychiatry Perspectives on 'Social Anxiety Disorder'*,
https://doi.org/10.1007/978-3-031-48707-1_5

desires of men'.[2] Drawing on the work of social theorist Patricia Hill Collins,[3] sociologists Laura T. Hamilton et al. write on the closely related notion of 'hegemonic femininities', which conceptualise the power relations underpinning these ideals. They explain: '*Hegemonic femininities are the most celebrated cultural ideals of womanhood in a given time and place that serve to uphold and legitimate all axes of oppression in the matrix of domination simultaneously.*'[4] Applying this to physical ideals specifically, feminist sociologist Meeta Jha points to 'beauty's imbrication in structural power relations of gender, race, nation, class, caste, inequality, and global culture'.[5]

In terms of physicality, which will be my concern in the first portion of this chapter, the 'western beauty aesthetic'[6] is found in 'young women with milky White skin, long blond hair, and slim figures'.[7] It is represented by the Barbie doll[8] and 'the blond, blue-eyed, white princess' of the Disney fairy tale.[9] Therefore, as Hamilton and colleagues point out, this 'culturally valued performanc[e] of femininity' is easiest for 'white, affluent, heterosexual, and cisgender'[10] women to enact.

On these feminine beauty ideals, Olivia told me that '[s]ince women are objectified in our patriarchal culture, girls and women face far more pressures than boys and men of being expected to always look a certain way'. Ellen likewise mentioned the 'pressure to look a certain way' and to 'conform to being a petite feminine lady'. Ellen's use of the word 'lady' is noteworthy, since, in addition to being a polite way of referring to a woman, it can also mean 'a woman of superior social position' and 'a woman of refinement and gentle manners'.[11] This suggests that race and class are inherent in the feminine ideal to which Ellen feels pressure to conform. Hamilton et al. elaborate on this in a manner pertinent to social anxiety, writing that '[t]he *interactional styles* of affluent white women [have] become coded as "classy" and styles of those who are less economically privileged or nonwhite as "trashy"'.[12]

The women with whom I talked not only discussed beauty ideals but related how these were intrinsic to their social anxiety. Ellen described her social anxiety as 'fear of being judged' and being 'about how I look'. She expanded on this, telling me, '[T]hat's why I'm anxious going somewhere where I don't look like what I think I should look like.' Olivia also described feeling 'self-conscious and hyper-conscious of my appearance', telling me, 'I feel more comfortable speaking on the phone than speaking face-to-face where I know that a judgement is being formed about me and how I look.' Likewise, Phoebe remembered a point in her life several years ago when

> I just felt really like just disgusting [...] like I was just the ugliest thing ever [...] so I guess that in itself is social anxiety, isn't it? Because it—I would feel really anxious in social situations because I would feel like people were looking at me.

At the time of writing, feminine beauty ideals are increasingly promulgated through social media. Criminology scholar Valerie Steeves makes the concurrent point that social media entails 'a clear and vigorously enforced set of social rules about acceptable ways of being a girl'.[13] This strikes a chord with Ellen's testimony, wherein she described how young women use social media:

> [I]t's the influencers as well, like, everyone is like, 'I need to get this, I need to look like this person.' I'm like, 'Oh, just look like yourself.' [...] They are told how to dress [...] that's why everyone—you go outside and everyone looks the same because it's social media.

Moreover, Steeves postulates that women's self-portrayal on social media is constrained in a manner which echoes the 'no-win' situations in which women find themselves in the workplace, wherein they must walk the fine line between being 'too feminine' and 'not feminine enough'. Social media is therefore

> [A] place where girls are open to criticism because they are [...] too made up, not made up enough, expose too much cleavage (and are therefore 'sluts'), don't expose enough cleavage, have too many friends (and are therefore 'desperate'), and/or don't have enough friends (and are therefore 'losers').[14]

Joan C. Chrisler and Ingrid Johnston-Robledo write on this delicate balance in observing that women's bodies must be 'beautiful (but not look like they tried too hard to achieve their beauty), sexy (but not slutty), pure (but not prudish) [and] slender (but curvy in the right places)'.[15] However, the double-bind which women face is more encompassing, for writer Chimamanda Ngozi Adichie describes girls' socialisation thus: 'We say to girls, you can have ambition, but not too much. You should aim to be successful, but not too successful.'[16] Likewise, implicit in Steeves's discussion is the need to cultivate an online image that is 'just right'.[17] Failure to achieve this can often result in 'harsh judgment'[18]—a nightmarish prospect for the already socially anxious woman, and I daresay a prospect which might nudge even the most confident of women into experiencing *some* social anxiety.

Building on the words of Adichie, the right kind of image is not restricted to the body's stylisation, but incorporates enacting 'highly gendered behavioural norms'.[19] This suggests that the regulation of appropriate femininity extends *beyond* appearance. As Hamilton and colleagues note, feminine beauty comprises 'embodiment, adornment, and deportment'.[20] And Deliovsky explains that 'a uniform social requirement of white women's acceptable *conduct* is their conformity to normative white femininity'.[21] Bringing this to bear online, social media presents a need for young women to be 'very careful' about how they represent themselves.[22] That is, non-conformance with '"appropriate" femininity'[23] engenders the risk of being unable to attain peer approval: something which Steeves argues 'plays an inordinately important role' in girls' socialisation.[24]

What is more, both on social media and off, a woman's appearance and body is used to garner all manner of facts about her character and personality. Chrisler and Johnston-Robledo allude to this being particularly prominent in women with intersecting identities, for '[p]eople are evaluated differently on the basis of information gleaned from observations of their bodies [and are] treated differently (e.g., racism, ageism, lookism, sizeism)'.[25] Art critic John Berger also comments on the importance of appearance in remarking that how a woman appears to others, especially men, 'is of crucial importance for what is normally thought of as the success of her life'.[26] And Susie Orbach writes that '[t]his emphasis on presentation as the central aspect of a woman's existence makes her extremely self-conscious'[27]—or, we might say, socially anxious. Author and academic Deborah L. Rhode succinctly sums up the significance of appearance thus:

> Beginning at birth, those who are viewed as physically appealing are also more likely to be viewed as smart, likeable and good. The ridicule and ostracism that unattractive children experience can result in lower self-confidence and social skills, which leads to further disadvantages later in life. Appearance also influences judgements about competence and job performance, which, in turn, affect income and status. Résumés get a less favorable assessment when they are thought to belong to less attractive individuals. These individuals are also less likely to get hired and promoted, and they earn lower salaries [...] *Women face greater pressures than men to look attractive and pay greater penalties for falling short.*[28]

While women face harsh penalties for *not* reaching the ideal, the obverse of this is that there are rewards to be had if they *do* reach it. On this point, Jha explains how skin-lightening and cosmetic surgery are ways in which

> [W]omen try to transform their physical appearance in order to increase their racial and beauty capital and access labor and marriage markets more successfully. In this way they may be able to reduce the effects of sexism, classism, and racism by gaining economic and cultural mobility. Women of color and working-class white women's desire for middle-class white beauty is founded rationally in their desire to surpass racial and working-class penalties.[29]

Jha's key contention is that women's striving towards the beauty ideal, to lessen the degree to which they are subject to structural inequalities, is quite logical. Following Rhode, women's fears about *not* reaching the ideal are equally logical, for failing to match up incurs barriers to success in a myriad of domains. One such domain is interpersonal relationships, and this is something Orbach addresses more directly. That is, 'Girls [...] seek connection with others and learn that this connection, especially with men, depends on the acceptability of their bodies.'[30] Farah's account strongly resonated with Orbach's tenet, for she spoke of a previous romantic partner: '[T]hat person didn't continue his relationship with me [...] I thought that it might be related to my appearance [...] because he was in [a] relationship with [an]other person, and [...] she's more beautiful than me.'

Having established the enormity of that which rests on women's physicality, as well as their self-portrayal more broadly, I wish to draw the reader's attention to one element of the *DSM-5*'s diagnostic criteria for SAD. That is, '[m]arked fear or anxiety about one or more social situations in which the individual is exposed to possible scrutiny by others'. This 'fear or anxiety' must be 'out of proportion to the actual threat posed by the social situation and to the sociocultural context'.[31] But given that women's successful performance of femininity is not only a gateway to success in multiple spheres, and there are tangible penalties if she should fall short, I ask: is her fear or anxiety about others' evaluations ever really 'out of proportion'?

This question develops an additional dimension if we consider Rhode's contention that appearance is seen to reflect personality traits. Olivia made a related, but slightly different, point in expressing that a woman's appearance reflects her 'worth and value', both in the eyes of 'individuals in their lives and by society and media at large'. Women then internalise this and 'their self-worth becomes based on their looks'. Feminist philosopher Sandra Lee Bartky makes a concordant point in stating that '[t]he sense of oneself as a [...] valuable individual is tied [...] to the sense of how one is perceived'.[32] Considering the significance that society attaches to a woman's appearance, her self-worth may become tied to how well others perceive her as reaching feminine beauty ideals.

We have thus far seen what the beauty ideal looks like and touched upon the axes of structural power which underpin it. But it has another feature: its elusiveness.[33] Chrisler and Johnston-Robledo liken striving towards it as 'a doomed project',[34] while Bartky describes it as 'a "setup": it requires such radical and extensive measures of bodily transformation that virtually every woman who gives herself to it is destined in some degree to fail'.[35] Bartky contends that this failure fosters shame[36] and erodes women's sense of value.[37] In keeping with Olivia's narrative, it promotes low self-worth and, echoing participants' narratives in Chap. 3, feelings of inadequacy. The prospect of facing these distressing emotions is likely to induce anxiety which might be tamped down if women, as Olivia tells us, spend 'lots of time on their appearance'.

In discussing how women spend their time, sociologist Arlie Hochschild's 1989 work *The Second Shift* becomes salient. Premised on case studies of two-job heterosexual couples, Hochschild opens the book by drawing on prior studies[38] in order to '[a]d[d] together the time it takes to do a paid job, housework, and child care'.[39] In so doing, Hochschild estimates that 'women worked roughly fifteen hours longer each week than men. Over a year, they worked an *extra month of twenty-four hour days.* Over a dozen years, it was an extra year of twenty four hour days'.[40] She continues:

> Most women without children spend much more time than men on housework; with children, they devote more time to caring for both house and children. Just as there is a wage gap between men and women in the workplace, there is a 'leisure gap' between them at home. Most women work one shift at the office or factory and a 'second shift' at home.[41]

Building on Hochschild's concept of the second shift, feminist writer Naomi Wolf dubs the time that women spend beautifying their bodies the 'third shift'.[42] While Hochschild notes that women are more likely to do 'jobs that fix them into a rigid routine',[43] such as cooking and cleaning, I propose that the third shift goes a step further, for beauty work is not a daily one-and-done job. Rather, it is a continuous and unrelenting process of maintenance, checking, and self-monitoring. And as Hochschild observes that 'women more often do two things at once—for example, write checks and return phone calls—vacuum and keep an eye on a three-year-old',[44] I note that these simultaneous tasks will also occur against a backdrop of beauty work. What is more, the labour that the third shift entails is often hidden. As Chrisler and Johnston-Robledo point out,

> [I]t is difficult to know exactly what types of beauty work other women do and how long it takes them to do it, so women may worry that they are not doing enough or that it takes them much longer than it takes other women to look their best.[45]

As such, not only does failing to *meet* the beauty ideal stoke feelings of low self-worth and inadequacy, but so too might the concern that one is not striving towards it in the correct, or most efficient, way.

The 'third shift' therefore exemplifies how beauty ideals function to discipline women's bodies and behaviours—a point which Bartky makes in her feminist reading of Michel Foucault's *Discipline and Punish*. In this opus, Foucault coins the term 'docile bodies' in describing our disciplinary society. To illustrate this concept, he tells us that in pre-modernity, men were chosen as soldiers based on pre-existing traits. By contrast, modernity saw the soldier first being chosen and then being 'constructed' into a 'machine' that exhibits the desired traits such that society's requirements are met.[46] He continues: 'A body is docile that may be subjected, used, transformed and improved';[47] the body is 'an object and target of power'.[48]

Bartky however holds that Foucault does not devote enough attention to the *female* docile body.[49] In exploring this, she tells us that, at her time of writing (1998), the trend for women's bodies is 'of a slimness bordering on emaciation'.[50] She nuances this point by noting that 'the current fitness movement has permitted women to develop more muscular strength and endurance than was heretofore allowed; indeed, images of women have begun to appear in the mass media that seem to eroticize this new muscularity'.[51] Bartky's words were prophetic, for the ideal feminine body—in much the same way as personality style—has come to incorporate some traditionally masculine elements, such as muscularity.[52] Writing in 2018, scholar Emily T. Troscianko termed this the 'bodybuilding-lite ideal' exemplified by 'the "toned" female with visible abdominals, pronounced glutes, and large breasts'.[53]

A rise in 'gym culture'[54] has likely nudged the development of the ideal in this direction and, like the ideals which came before, it is enmeshed with the popularisation of social media. Gym culture's growth has also entailed a proliferation of 'healthism', that is, 'the sociocultural pressure to strive to achieve perfect health and fitness'.[55] Chrisler and Johnston-Robledo call healthism 'another body project often taken up by women, especially those of higher socioeconomic classes',[56] thereby speaking to the beauty ideal's imbuement with class privilege. They go on to explain that '[b]ecause health and fitness are often confounded with beauty, healthism provides cover for beauty work (e.g., "I'm exercising not for vanity but for my health.")'.[57] This further occludes the time that women spend on the third shift.

The imbrications of social media with gym culture, healthism, and bodily ideals came to the fore when I interviewed Ellen. She told me, 'I think because I do follow all of that on Instagram [...] I am like, "[...] she can do a pull up. Why can't I do a pull up?"' Ellen however seemed cognizant that her social media use fuelled her having high, and perhaps unrealistic, expectations of herself. Following her previous remark, she said, '[A]ctually, she's like 5 foot and really tiny and I'm not, so I've got a lot more weight to lift.' Ellen went on to propose how she might achieve a healthier body image and higher self-esteem, stating, 'I reckon if I removed all of that and all I followed was like fat activists like Lizzo or like Tess Holliday, I think I'd be fine, I think I would stop caring.' Ellen's acknowledgement of the potential harms of consuming mainstream social media content has much in common with Steeves's research on social media use in young women. One of Steeves's participants 'felt that the ubiquitous presence of diet ads, weight loss tips, and other "beauty aids," on social media, as well as pages posted by models and clothing companies, created an overwhelming desire to "change my body"'.[58]

On the other hand, Ellen alluded to social media being a means by which body positivity could be promoted and different physiques celebrated. To focus on the figures that Ellen mentioned, Tess Holliday made headlines in 2015 for becoming the largest plus-sized model to be contracted by a mainstream agency[59] and she also founded the online body positivity movement *EffYourBeautyStandards*.[60] Ellen told me about Lizzo:

> [S]he was in an interview where someone said to her like, 'Oh, you wouldn't look good skinny anyway,' she's like, 'Honey, I look good any size.' [...] [S]he's a rapper and a singer [...] basically like a fat activist and she's just really cool.

Despite Ellen demonstrating insight into how she could improve her body image and wellbeing by means of her social media use, I sensed reluctance in her to commit to what she was proposing. She seemed to harbour an unwillingness to renounce fully the body and lifestyle ideals espoused by the fitness and gym culture Instagram accounts in question. This sentiment is analogous to that of a number of women in the fat acceptance movement, and one which also strikes a chord with Ellen's narrative later on in this chapter: 'I'm totally smart and a feminist...and yet I want to be a waif.'[61]

As Bartky predicted, the body ideal has evolved beyond that of the waif such that it now features more muscularity. With that said, it is still, if not merely 'thin', characterised by low body fat. In order to achieve this, the majority of women will have to exercise. Moreover, as Bartky contends, most women will have to diet, which 'disciplines the body's hungers'.[62] The upshot of this is that diet and exercise serve to discipline the body, its size, and the space it takes up.

Taking up Space

Underlying many participants' discomfort with their body size was a reluctance to take up space. This was a recurring theme in Ellen's interview:

> I find myself trying to shrink myself and it's horrible [...] we're meant to care about our size and not taking up too much space [...] I'm always paranoid about my height. I'm like, 'I take up too much space for a woman.'

Phoebe also spoke about taking up space and recalled one instance in particular: 'I remember once I had a massive panic attack because I was having to budge through chairs [...] I got really anxious that I wasn't going to fit.' Bartky describes comparable accounts from women in her own work as being indicative of deep shame[63] and 'a measure of the extent to which all women have internalized patriarchal standards of bodily acceptability'.[64]

But it is not only women's body *size* which is significant to their taking up space. Indeed, Bartky notes that women's body *comportment* is more restricted than men's. Referencing political scientist Iris Young, she proposes that '[w]oman's body language speaks eloquently, though silently, of her subordinate status in a hierarchy of gender'.[65] Feminist photographer Marianne Wex's work, wherein she examines photographs of men and women in public areas, corroborates this.[66] Wex found that, when sitting and waiting for trains, women tend to sit with their legs together and their hands in their laps, apparently aiming to take up as little space as they can. This links to Amy's testimony insofar as she spoke about

> [F]eeling like I'm not allowed to take up space and that I should be conscientious of the space that I'm taking up [...] I definitely see that as a gendered problem [...] the female programming is that like low-key instinct not to take up space.

Phoebe's testimony was similar, since she stated that 'you're told to like shrink in—both physically and mentally, I think, and then that plays out in like your social life'. Lily Myers's poem 'Shrinking Women'[67] encapsulates the gendering of taking up space which Phoebe, Ellen, and Amy all describe. Therein, Myers imagines saying to her brother, '[Y]ou have been taught to grow out, I have been taught to grow in.' Myers's words follow Wex's study: when sitting and waiting for trains, usually men were found to sit with their arms out to their sides and their legs apart, apparently unconcerned with taking up space.[68] This tendency had not escaped the notice of Amy, since she described 'the men around me unabashedly taking up space'. She also shared how this made her feel: '[I]t makes me really mad [...] because I don't have that privilege [...] it's almost a jealously thing, like, "How dare you take up all of this space [...]?"' Amy's remarks allude to public spaces being implicitly male—a patent manifestation of which is women's daily experiences of enduring street harassment.[69]

Ellen's experience is also relevant to the gendering of space, for she told me that she is 'scared of the "man area" at the gym'. In his work on gender and gym culture, sociologist Thomas Johansson notes that as late modernity has seen the body become a project, the gym has become a place where 'the body is cultivated'.[70] Johansson's work links with Ellen's narrative in that he describes the gym as 'a gendered space, where certain body techniques and locations are related to the female body and others with the male body [...] where the bodybuilding culture meets the aerobics culture'.[71] Ellen's apprehension about entering the 'man area' of the gym could thus be construed as unease about transgressing gender norms by entering an implicitly male space. Indeed, Johansson tells us that 'women often feel like aliens when stepping into the male space'.[72] Ria gave an example which resonates with Johansson's latter remark, but on the gendering of space in a figurative sense. She described standing up to deliver a speech, an arguably masculine activity demanding assertiveness and aplomb. This scenario precipitated in her the 'feeling like you don't have any ownership in the space you're in'.

Following on from this, Amy connected taking up space to her social anxiety, telling me, '[M]y social anxiety makes me even more aware of the space I take up.' She then pondered: '[I]s my social anxiety spatial awareness part of or driven by the female programming that says "don't take up space"? They're probably interconnected.' Furthermore, she elaborated on exactly *why* the gendering of taking up space irked her:

> [Y]ou'd be frustrated if somebody was standing in your way, right? And then you'd be more frustrated if that person was a man who was clearly like completely blanking on how he's affecting other people. And then you'd be more frustrated when you realise that that's a systematic problem [...] That's how society has taught men that they're allowed to be. Or, more specifically, that's how society's taught women they're *not* allowed to be. And then it goes, 'Oh, actually, is the man doing the wrong here or has society done me the disservice of convincing me I have to be aware of the space I take up?'

Amy's recognition that the gendering of taking up space is a systemic problem compounds her distress surrounding this issue. I want now to bring in Derald Wing Sue's microaggressions, of which the gendering of public space and the (in)ability for women to take up space are examples. As well as featuring in women's day-to-day lives, microaggressions operate 'on a systemic and macro level'.[73] They are painful reminders of greater structural inequalities precisely because they arise from the very same institutional biases that 'affect [...] quality of life and standard of living' and 'den[y] equal access and opportunities in education, employment, and health care [...] for marginalized groups in our society'.[74] Is Ria's experience of being undermined in the workplace not a reminder that women still earn, on average, 9% less than men for doing the same job?[75] Does street harassment not arise from the same misogyny which leads to one in five women over the age of 16 being sexually assaulted?[76] These pairs of phenomena lend themselves to Gloria Anzaldúa's *la facultad*—'[T]he capacity to see in surface phenomena the meaning of deeper realities'[77]—to which the marginalised are more sensitised. As the gendering of taking up space angers Amy, Ellen alluded to street harassment affecting her analogously: '[I]t constantly happens to women. Like, you will be cat called [...] it's an everyday battle, so therefore why would you not internalise [...] take that with you and worry about it the next day? Because it's every day.' To Ellen's point, that we cannot exist undisturbed in public spaces is a bleak reminder that *all* women are supposed to exist solely for men's consumption.

The gendering of public space and the associated imperative that women *not* take up space were key in participants' experiences of social anxiety insofar as they stoked self-consciousness and concerns about others' perceptions. But it would be remiss to discuss taking up space and gloss over a vital metric which is related so closely to it: weight.

Weight

Weight warrants a subsection of its own both due to its prominence in participants' testimonies and its being bound more strongly to oppression than other metrics of body size, such as height. This was evidenced when I asked Daniella if her concern with her appearance was related to weight, to which she replied, 'Yeah, of course, absolutely [...] [I]t's the thing underlying everything.' While thinness in women is prized, conversely, as sociologists Ariane Prohaska and Jeannine A. Gailey tell us, 'The oppression of fat people is built into institutions, pervades the cultural landscape, and affects the relationships and perceptions of people of size.'[78] In line with this, academics Helen Hester and Caroline Walters describe 'a contemporary cultural landscape that is openly hostile towards fat people and their perceived social and aesthetic transgressions'.[79] As such, it is perhaps no surprise that discrimination against people who fit the criteria for obesity has been called 'an acceptable prejudice'.[80] Indeed, Prohaska and Gailey cite a body of work which claims that fat people face barriers to higher pay and promotion in the workplace;[81] draws attention to how they are oftentimes portrayed in a negative manner in television and film;[82] and posits that fat defendants in the courtroom are subject to weight bias.[83] In particular, fat *women*, they hold, are 'not perceived as believable victims of intimate partner violence or sexual assault because they do not fit the stereotype of a "typical" (thin or attractive) victim'.[84] Moreover, they argue that fat women 'are less likely than their thin counterparts to be labeled as desirable relationship or sexual partners'.[85]

Academic Noortje van Amsterdam's work follows this in that it theorises the intersection of body size with other axes of oppression. In particular, van Amsterdam contends that evaluations as to whether somebody actually *is* fat depend heavily on their gender: 'As a man, he is just a big dude; as a woman, she is revoltingly fat.'[86] Moreover, she finds that 'fat men can find ways to construct a positive fat identity' by drawing on 'representations of male bodies as big and powerful'. Yet, 'These constructions of positive fat identity tend not to be available to women, since they are incongruent with (heterosexual White) femininity.'[87] It seems, therefore, that the fatphobia with which society is awash is uniquely poisonous towards women, with thinness forming a cornerstone of the feminine bodily ideal.

Ellen's account drew links with this in that she related how losing weight had inched her closer to this ideal:

> [W]hen I was dumped, I lost like 2 stone really quickly, but that was just the fact that I was sad and I couldn't eat [...] I got to a point where I was like, 'I look great,' and [...] all of my friends were like, 'Yeah, but you're sad, you're really sad.' And I was like, 'But I'm skinny!'

Ellen's sentiment here reflects society's tacit viewpoint that a woman's thin body trumps all, even her mental wellbeing. This brings to mind one of the fat acceptance movement's tenets, commonly deployed in response to expressed 'concern' regarding the health ramifications of being a given weight. Fat activist Victoria Welsby sums this up thus: '[I]f you actually cared about fat people's health then you would care about their mental health.'[88] Welsby raises a relevant point: Prohaska and Gailey put forth that, for fat people, '[T]he impact of stigma can lead to feelings of shame, isolation, lower self-esteem, poor body image, and an increased risk of other mental health issues.'[89]

Likewise, the prospect of being perceived as fat could well promote feeling ill at ease, especially for women. This was certainly the case for Phoebe, who shared the following anecdote: '[W]hen I went to university I became really like aware of my weight and very like self-conscious.' Quite literally, the thin ideal engenders the threat of one's body not fitting in. This is because, as van Amsterdam explains, '[D]ominant discourses on beauty and health co-construct a body hierarchy which positions slender people as the norm (the unmarked position) and fat people as deviant or dissonant (the marked position).'[90] Normativity pervaded Chap. 3, wherein belonging was a common thread in participants' experiences of social anxiety. This is a theme which is also salient for the body. That is, if we are to follow Susie Orbach, belonging is key in many women's experiences of Anorexia Nervosa—they may at first have pursued 'thinness in order to feel acceptable. Acceptance may have at first meant fitting in'.[91] Ria's story meshes with Orbach's tenet, for she cited being an outlier in a statistical sense as having precipitated her eating problems:

> [W]hen I thought my eating disorder started, I was about nine years old. And we were in a maths class, and we were doing scatter plots. And we were plotting height vs. weight. And I was a little bit of an outlier [...] I remember people pointing at the outlier, and, 'Who's that?' [...] I was like, 'Ok, maybe I could do with losing a few pounds.'

My own school years were peppered with experiences like Ria's. One which stands out in my mind is an Information Technology lesson when I was around eight years old. We had been tasked with filling databases with data and one of the metrics the teacher had chosen was waist circumference. After the initial embarrassment I felt when my measurement was larger than most of my classmates', I remember thinking, much like Ria, that I needed to lose weight—a thought which would accompany me well into adulthood.

Daniella spoke about having this same thought herself as a young adult. Upon moving to the UK from continental Europe at age 18, she related that: 'I didn't know anyone [...] I kind of felt like [...] I had to show a better appearance of myself [...] So, at that time, I started losing a lot of weight.' We can better understand Daniella's experience if we examine it through Deaux and Greenwood's work on gender and immigration.[92] That is, 'In Western cultures, immigrants are measured against white, Eurocentric, and secular norms, and experience pressure to conform to these norms.'[93] In turn, 'Immigrants who closely "fit" the social representations of men and women in the host culture are likely to find a smoother road to integration than those whose traditions, norms, and occupations mark them as different or "Other".'[94] As such, Daniella seems to be suggesting that portraying herself in the best light—adhering to Anglo-American feminine norms by possessing a thin body—would better equip her to secure new relationships in the UK. This strongly echoes Orbach's argument that '[g]irls [...] seek connection with others and learn that this connection, especially with men, depends on the acceptability of their bodies'.[95] Indeed, many participants described a link between their bodies and their relationships, not least Daniella:

> [T]he reason why [...] I don't want to see people is because I don't want them to see me at this size [...] when I was trying to like rationalise the fact that I didn't want to meet people, it was like, 'Would that be different if I were thin?' And the answer is, 'Yes [...] it wouldn't bother me as much.' [...] [T]hat's why I'm refusing to go home [...] I haven't seen my family in a long time [...] especially my mum's side, they would say things [...] they're [...] very upfront. So it'll be like, 'Oh, you chunked up.'

Whereas Daniella told me how she *imagines* her family will react to her body, Phoebe told me about comparable exchanges which *actually came to pass* with her relatives:

> [T]hat side of my family are like massively like fat-phobic [...] my uncle said to me, '[...] [Y]ou've got a real blubbery layer and you really need to like get rid of it.' [...] I remember asking my cousin, '[...] [D]o you think I do?' [...] and she was like, '[...] [Y]ou do [...] but you can like get rid of it in this way.'

Phoebe's and Daniella's accounts painfully resonate with my own experience, most acute in childhood and adolescence but persisting into adulthood. On the one hand, we have the unrelenting criticism and commentary on my body shape and size with interludes of comparing and contrasting with various others—friends, relatives, acquaintances, celebrities—peppered with bouts of scolding and shaming. But on the other hand we have the praise and admiration, most prominent on the two occasions when I lost so much weight that my periods stopped for the best part of a year: 'You look *great*!'; 'How did you do it?'; and, ironically, being told by an acquaintance I had not seen in a while that it was 'good to see me looking so well'. Phoebe's, Daniella's, and my own experiences gel with Bartky's observation that '"people" – friends and casual acquaintances alike – act to enforce prevailing standards of body size'.[96]

The remarks from these 'people', such as Phoebe's uncle, suggest that Daniella is perhaps rational in fearing her family's reaction to changes in her body, and, in turn, how this will make her feel. Indeed, Phoebe remembered how she herself felt following her uncle's remarks, after which she sought reassurance from her cousin: '[T]hat made me really sad because I was like, [...] "I just really needed you to be kind in that moment because I felt really vulnerable", I was only like eighteen.' For my part, it is not necessarily remarks about my body *per se* which can be so gutting (though they can and often are). Rather, in the spirit of Anzaldúa's *la facultad*, my distress results from an awareness of what the pervasiveness of these unsolicited remarks signifies: the mandate to adhere to an ideal which not only upholds my own oppression but is deleterious to my health and wellbeing; that in others' eyes—and perhaps my own—my worth is contingent on the degree to which I meet this ideal; and, following Rhode, the very real penalties I face if I am seen to fall short.[97]

Conversely, recall that Jha outlines the rewards to be reaped if women succeed in reaching the (thin) ideal.[98] In keeping with this, Daniella reflected on the potential benefits of losing weight: '[T]hey always say, "Oh, if you lose weight, it's not going to solve your problems." It might solve a few of mine. Because a lot of mine are related to weight.' Orbach speaks to this dominant cultural message in observing that '[g]irls from the age of nine right through to women in their sixties have absorbed the message that they *can* solve emotional problems, sexual problems, family problems, relationship problems, work problems—all through the transformation of their body size'.[99] This may well be true for Daniella, since some of her problems seem to arise not from her weight *per se*, but from how others—'people'[100]—react to it. Ellen made an analogous point about her height:

> I'm 6 foot [...] I've internalised the fact that I'm like, 'Oh, I'm masculine, people are going to look at me because I look like a man, they're going to be judging me for my height and then [...] I'll get called big.'

Daniella's expectation of how others will react to her weight is remarkably similar to Phoebe's actual experience and, I wager, most other women's—it certainly is to mine. Day after day, we are exposed to the commentary of 'people',[101] as Phoebe described: '[F]eeling like people are talking about your body, or like, "Oh, you've lost weight, she's put on weight," that kind of thing.' The prescience of Daniella's prediction derives from her being immersed in this milieu but, more directly, it is informed by her prior experience. Specifically, she told me: 'I was always chunky, I mean, as a kid: the reason why I was bullied.' Given this, her concerns about how others will perceive her body seem quite justifiable. This calls into question whether the facet of women's social anxiety which centres on the fear of their bodies being negatively evaluated is best framed as a mental disorder. Would it not be better framed as a rational response to how society treats non-normative, especially fat, women's bodies?

Following on from this, women may seek, understandably so, to change their bodies to fit the thin ideal. One of the means by which they may strive to do this is through the modification of food intake. Like myself, Daniella, Ria, and Phoebe had all experienced eating problems which, for each of them, originated from wanting to change how they look in light of concerns about others' perceptions.

Eating Problems

Phoebe's experiences with eating and exercising featured prominently in her narrative. She began by telling me:

> It was never diagnosed but I think I probably had some sort of eating disorder[102] where I would like exercise kind of like compulsively [...] I would eat but in a way where only if I could counterbalance it with exercise [...] so I was like that for a few years [...] I never had a day off, for months. [...] I would run like a half marathon every day.

While Phoebe's account draws links with the diagnostic criteria for Anorexia Nervosa—namely, 'strict rituals around eating'[103] and 'energy intake restriction'[104]—a large proportion of women could be said, to varying degrees, to restrict their intake in light of cultural ideals about thinness. Indeed, social psychologist Helen Malson tells us that dieting is now 'more prevalent and therefore more "normal" or normative than *non*-dieting amongst women and girls'.[105] Following Chloë Taylor, who tells us that traditionally feminine traits are deemed to be abnormal when they are exaggerated,[106] it appears that energy intake restriction is deemed to be pathological only when in the extreme. In other words, women must restrict energy intake, but not too much: yet another double bind.

In the spirit of conceptualising women's eating problems as comprehensible responses to their socialisation, I wish to remind the reader of participants' earlier allusions to weight loss being a means by which to moderate the impressions of others. Social anxiety then appears to be intertwined with eating problems insofar as both forms of mental distress often concern achieving a normative body. Quite literally, this means fitting in and, by extension, acceptance. Given this, the *DSM-5*'s conceptualisation of Anorexia Nervosa as merely 'an intense fear of gaining weight or becoming fat'[107] is wildly reductive. No attention is devoted to why women might have this very rational fear: namely, bearing witness to how society treats fat (women's) bodies. In addition to the work of fat studies scholars cited earlier on in the chapter, a further example is found in the relatively recent ban of the Reddit community 'fat people hate'.[108] Moreover, psychoanalyst Marilyn Lawrence cites a study by Lenore F. Monello and Jean Mayer in which the authors contend that 'the prejudice against fat people is similar to that directed against certain racial minorities'.[109] Author Kathleen LeBesco however notes that a key difference between the two is that 'there's little in the way of public norms to keep people from expressing anti-fat sentiment in public'.[110] Lawrence expounds upon Monello and Mayer's study thus:

> [F]at people themselves suffer the same damage to their self-esteem and share the same resistance to achievement as that found amongst racial minorities who are subject to social hatred and discrimination. The effect of these negative images and associations with fat is to make us overvalue thinness.[111]

This overvaluing gives rise to vigilance: thinness must be achieved and, once achieved, maintained. It follows that control, or losing it, featured in many participants' testimonies. Daniella shared her experience: '[W]hen I had Anorexia, the only satisfying thing about it was that I was in control [...] when I binge [eat] I don't have measure, I don't have control, I lose control and that makes me super anxious.' Although Ria spoke of Bulimia Nervosa, her account told a similar story: 'I guess the eating, and as it started, I think it probably was a control thing.' While the overvaluing of thinness may give rise to the need for control, Lawrence's conceptualisation of the anorexic experience as the 'control paradox' provides another explanation. She describes this as

> [V]ery powerful control which anorexics exert in the area of food and weight and their own experience of themselves as utterly out of control. Anorexics are attempting to solve the problem of their own powerlessness and denigration as women by engaging in an internal struggle for self-control.[112]

Lawrence contends that women feel unable to control their environment, which sees control then turn inward:[113] '[W]omen are encouraged to locate any difficulties they feel inside themselves rather than in the world'[114]—a standpoint congruent with the individual pathology model. Author Morag MacSween conceptualises Anorexia Nervosa similarly, describing it as 'an indirect and individualized response to a *social* issue'.[115] Applying this to participants' stories, we might construe a woman's eating problems as her struggle to mould her body to the norm—and hence evade negative evaluation—since she cannot control the mandate that she adhere to the norm; the ramifications if she falls short; the very existence of the norm or its nature.

In discussing eating problems thus far, I have focused on energy *restriction*. But this was but one element which featured in participants' accounts. As Daniella earlier alluded to her experience with binge eating, she went on to describe it thus:

> I started what's my now Binge Eating Disorder. So that's a massive part of my mental health [...] it's the main thing that contributes to my mood swings. So, if I'm eating right, my mood is up, if I'm eating wrong, my mood is low.

Just as a woman's personality, emotions, and appearance can all be 'right' or 'wrong', so too, it seems, can the way that she eats. This draws links with the morality that is bestowed upon food,[116] something which Lawrence finds to be exemplified in the oft-repeated phrase 'it's illegal, it's immoral or it makes you fat'.[117] She continues: 'Self-denial in the area of food will therefore bring with it some fairly far-reaching moral kudos, and will be an indicator of moral worth.'[118] As such, being a good and attractive woman in our culture not only means having the right personality style and the right body but also—in a nod to my prior discussion of the expectation that women put others' needs before their own—the ability to deny oneself.[119] Failure on the part of women to exercise restraint in terms of their food intake is thus likely to invite negative judgement from others. The *DSM-5*'s diagnostic criteria for Anorexia Nervosa state that 'individuals may feel humiliated or embarrassed to be seen eating in public, as in social phobia'.[120] What this omits is that this concern is explicable if we consider the morality conferred on food. And somebody seen to be indulging, as opposed to restraining, their appetite is likely to be frowned upon[121]—especially if this person is a woman.[122]

As I ponder the morality of food, and, in turn, a thin body, the words of an old friend ring in my ears. Years ago, we were about to order food at a café, and she said, 'I think I'm going to have the kale—then I can feel virtuous.' Although this was likely said, at least partially, in jest, it speaks to the conflation of health with virtue. Daniella hinted at this in explaining to me why she wanted to lose weight from her, to my eye, already-slender frame: 'It's not just that I want to look thin, it's not just an appearance line, but it's a physical thing as well [...] it's health.' Peter Conrad suggests that 'health can be a moral discourse and the body a site for moral action'. Engaging in the pursuit of wellness, of which physical health and weight management is a part, 'becomes seen as a good in itself'.[123] And just as healthism 'provides an opportunity to blame and shame ill people who are perceived as not having "worked hard" enough to be healthy',[124] so too does it provide an opportunity to blame and shame people who are fat.

What is ironic about slenderness being tied to health is that, in order to attain the level of thinness required by the ideal, it is necessary for most women to diet—a state which Wolf calls 'semistarvation'.[125] Wolf cites a body of work which has linked 'chronic dieting' to 'irritability, poor concentration, anxiety, depression, apathy, lability of mood, fatigue and social isolation'.[126] Ria mentioned chronic hunger affecting women's emotional states in noticing how 'women seem to get "hangry" more than men do [...] is that the socialisation [...] the fact that women don't eat to be full?' Pertinent to Ria's observation is Wolf's citing of the Minnesota Starvation Experiment.[127] Headed by physiologist Ancel Keys and taking place between 1944 and 1945, the study took 36 men and, over a period of 24 weeks, reduced their caloric intake such that they lost an average of 25% of their bodyweight. Crucially, the study found that extended semistarvation caused depression and hysteria, with the majority of the participants experiencing high levels of mental distress.[128] This speaks to the embodied conceptualisation of women's social anxiety which was theorised in Chap. 3. Paradoxically, it also suggests that through engaging in chronic dieting to pursue the thin ideal—in order to fit in and hence mitigate social anxiety—women might actually render themselves *more* (socially) anxious than they otherwise would be.

On pursuing the thin ideal, Orbach characterises the body as key in the search for identity.[129] That is, the body is one's 'calling card, vested with showing the results of our hard work and watchfulness or, alternatively, our failure and sloth'.[130] On this point, Lawrence tells us that

> We behave as though the body is indeed the mirror of the soul. Fat people, simply by virtue of their shape and size, seem to be telling us that they are careless, indolent, lacking in self-control and even in sensitivity.[131]

Rosalind Gill argues that this is emblematic of postfeminist media culture, wherein the female body

> [I]s constructed as a window to the individual's interior life. For example, in Bridget Jones's Diary[132] when Bridget Jones smokes 40 cigarettes a day or consumes 'excessive' calories, we are invited to read this in psychological terms as indicative of her emotional breakdown.[133]

The link between women's bodies and their interior lives was present in Ellen's testimony, for she told me how women are 'surveyed on how we behave as well'. Gill elaborates on this, proposing that 'monitoring and surveying the self have long been requirements of the performance of successful femininity — with instruction in grooming, attire, posture, elocution and "manners" being "offered" to women to allow them to emulate more closely the upper-class white ideal'.[134] In the age of postfeminism, it seems that the requirement to regulate extends from the body to body comportment, behaviour, and character. Gill continues:

> [I]t is not only the surface of the body that needs ongoing vigilance — there is also the self: what kind of friend, lover, daughter, or colleague are you? Do you laugh enough? How well do you communicate? Have you got emotional intelligence? [...] the self has become a project to be evaluated, advised, disciplined and improved or brought 'into recovery'.[135]

As I theorised in Chap. 4 how current femininity views the *body* as a project, Gill articulates how this has bled through to encompass the whole self. Brumberg has written on this notion in analysing American girls' diaries from 1830–1990. She finds that, with time, girls' concerns with self-improvement shift, most markedly in the middle of the twentieth century, from the internal—they wanted to be 'more patient, kinder, gentler, more loving, more devoutly faithful, more trustworthy'—to the external—they 'wanted to become more attractive people, prettier and thinner'.[136] For these girls, 'The soul seems to have been replaced by the body as "the object of salvation".'[137] Following Gill, the second decade of the twenty-first century has *almost* seen this come full circle. Self-improvement once again concerns the self, not *instead of*, but *as well as* the body—it concerns women's whole embodied selves. One of the places where this most visibly plays out is on social media.

'Be the Best Version of Yourself'

The ubiquity of self-improvement discourses on social media came up when I was talking with Ria:

> Katie: [I]t's like continuous betterment […] 'Oh, you have to be the best version of yourself,' just like in—
>
> Ria: Oh! 'Be your best self,' I hate that! I hate that phrase! […] 'Be my best self.' Shut up! […] I think it's one of the worst—it—I think it epitomises what's terrible now.

Social media is teeming with the notion of being one's 'best self'. An archetypal post peddling this idea comprises a scenic background—perhaps a sunset or a meadow—overlain with an 'inspirational' quote such as, 'I'm working on myself, for myself, by myself',[138] or, '[Y]our biggest opponent is yourself.'[139] This rhetoric represents a shift from the idea that we should all strive to be like the 'influencer' on our Instagram feed—the white upper-class woman who embodies the feminine ideal—and a move towards the idea that we should strive to be 'the best version of ourselves'. A fictional and idealised image of ourselves is therefore evoked; and it is within reach, if only we put in the work. I am reminded here of the following quote, attributed to an anonymous source: 'Someone once told me the definition of hell: on your last day on earth, the person you could have become will meet the person you became.' Failure to measure up to this fanciful notion can only fuel feelings of inadequacy: feelings which were already so prominent in participants' narratives in Chap. 3. In turn, the prospect of not being our 'best selves' stokes the fear that others will look upon us unfavourably, per social anxiety, precisely because they encourage us to look upon *ourselves* unfavourably.

Personal betterment rhetoric has much in common with Harris's conceptualisation of modern-day femininity. Harris tells us that 'can-do' femininity has its beginnings in the 'grrrl' movement of the 1990s: '[I]ts punk philosophy of DIY (do it yourself) and individual responsibility for social change lent itself easily to its transformation into a discourse of choice and focus on the self.'[140] 'Girlpower' was inherent in this movement, and this incorporated ambition, confidence, outspokenness, self-belief and, most notably, 'power through and control over one's own identity invention and re-invention'.[141] The present-day feminine ideals with which social media is replete have continued to follow this trajectory insofar as they conceive of the self as a 'DIY project' on which a woman should work.[142]

Implicit in this rhetoric is the sentiment that what happens to us is completely and utterly under our control. Indeed, Shani Orgad notes that 'emphasis on individual responsibility gained particular currency in emerging postfeminist media discourses in the 1990s'.[143] Likewise, Gill puts forth that postfeminist discourses contain an 'emphasis upon empowerment and taking control that can be seen in talk shows, advertising and makeover shows'[144]—and, I argue, on social media. In being critical of the emphasis on self-determination, personal choice,[145] and women's being 'free to shape their own destiny',[146] I am not suggesting that women do not have agency. Rather, I am making the case that these self-betterment discourses promote the idea that if one only works hard enough to better oneself, one can achieve ***absolutely anything***, irrespective of structural inequalities. On this point, Gill argues that postfeminist discourses espouse '[t]he notion that all our practices are freely chosen' and that women are 'autonomous agents no longer constrained by any inequalities or power imbalances whatsoever'.[147] She continues: '[E]ven experiences of racism, homophobia or domestic violence are framed in exclusively personal terms in a way that turns the idea of the personal-as-political on its head.'[148]

The idealised version of the self, towards which women are relentlessly supposed to aspire, has been called 'a dangerous fiction'[149] by Angela McRobbie. Ria seemed to concur with this, for she pushed back against the demand that she cultivate an image of herself that is perfect to the extent of being non-human. In response to this demand, she told me: 'No. Sometimes, I want to sit in my pyjamas, with a big, fat ice cream.' Despite her apparent resistance, the pressure to be her 'best self' seemed inescapable for Ria, since she followed the above remark with 'I shouldn't care that people know that.'

As one's 'best self' incorporates all aspects of the self, including the corporeal, it is pertinent to explore Malson's exposition of humanistic discourse. This 'dictates that it is the inner self, an individual's character rather than their appearance, which is important and should be valued'.[150] With that said, Malson warns that this discourse 'does not necessarily lessen the imperative to be thin'[151] for women. Instead, it may 'result in a negative interpellation of the subject as irrational and superficial, as being too concerned with appearance'.[152] This creates a conflict: one wants to adhere to the bodily ideal, but, in so wanting, feels guilty. I alluded to a conflict of this kind earlier in exploring Ellen's social media use, and it is to her words that I now return. She told me, '[I]t's weird, because I don't care what other people think, I care—I'm like, "Oh, I want to look like that." But [...] *why* do I want to look like that?' For Ellen, this tension extended to the newer, more fringe phenomenon of body positivity:

> I constantly battle with myself, I'm like, 'All bodies are amazing,' and I'm like, 'Apart from mine.' [...] I've never ever looked at anyone else and thought, 'You shouldn't wear that.' [...] But to myself, I'm like, 'Hmm... You can't wear that.'

While Ellen acknowledged some of the harms that the existence of a feminine bodily ideal brings, she experienced difficulty in, to quote psychologists Ngaire Donaghue and Anne Clemitshaw, 'resisting the "thin ideal" that has become such a normative requirement of successful western femininity'[153] when it came to her *own* body. Donaghue and Clemitshaw note a comparable feeling among women within the fat acceptance movement, which I previously cited: 'I'm totally smart and a feminist...and yet I want to be a waif.'[154]

Ellen went on to detail how she experiences an analogous conflict about attitudes towards food and the expectation that women self-deny:

> I find myself challenging people every day that are like, 'Oh, I'm not going to—' I'm like, 'No food is bad.' [...] [E]ven though in my own head I'll go home and be like, 'I can't have a bite of that.'

Ria also articulated a tension regarding food, though hers was slightly different:

> [O]ne thing I've noticed [...] is that I enjoy the idea that people think I eat a lot [...] you know the whole thing of like, eating a nice big portion in front of people and they're like, 'Ooh, how do you stay so slim?' [...] 'How amazing!' And I think part of me really liked that.

Alongside this, Ria experienced guilt about creating an enviable, but perhaps unrealistic, image of herself as a woman who eats a lot without gaining weight, since she also said: 'I'm going to try and stop myself [...] It's stupid, I shouldn't do it [...] it's not good.'

Ellen's and Ria's experiences of conflicts and tensions harbour another phenomenon: self-critique. This ran through other participants' narratives, both implicitly and explicitly, and will thus be the target of my analysis in what follows. However, to lay the required groundwork for this, the necessary precursors need to be explored: namely, the notion that women are watched and, in turn, come to watch themselves.

Being Watched

Many participants related their own experiences of being watched, and explained how such experiences triggered their social anxiety:

> Ellen: I have that panic of, 'Oh, that's why I'm being looked at,' and that will make me anxious.
>
> Olivia: I don't like being looked at because I over-worry about how I'm being perceived.
>
> Phoebe: I would feel really anxious in social situations because I would feel like people were looking at me.

Phoebe elaborated on her experience, telling me about her time at university:

> [I]f there's someone that I'm embarrassed of my behaviour from when I was younger [...] guys I've slept with or whatever [...] I would get so anxious about seeing them [...] to the point where I would like avoid leaving my flat, if I could, because I would get worried [...] in case I saw them.

While Phoebe detailed feeling apprehensive about *seeing* certain people around her city, we might also read this as her fear of *being seen* and, in turn, judged unfavourably. On this notion, Chrisler and Johnston-Robledo call attention to '[t]he trendiness of revealing clothing and the ubiquity of cell phone cameras [which] mean that girls' and women's bodies are nearly always in view and subject to the judgments of others'.[155] Ellen resisted this trend, telling me: 'That's why I really like Billie Eilish for girls [...] She only wears really, really baggy, bright clothes [...] so as the media can't get pictures of her to scrutinise her body.'

Orbach has also commented on women's visibility, describing how social media can be used to 'post unflattering pictures of individuals which are then "snarked" and negatively commented on'.[156] In the UK, this assumes the form of 'Spotted' pages on Facebook,[157] where users can anonymously post candid photographs of students on which other users can comment. As *Everyday Sexism Project* founder Laura Bates writes, these comments usually take the form of evaluating the (female) subject's appearance and are often both highly sexualized, objectifying, and sexist.[158] As a second-year undergraduate back in 2012, I unhappily chanced upon my own university's 'Spotted' page which, sure enough, assumed the form that Bates describes. I can still remember the unease and vigilance I felt whilst walking around campus thereafter.

A kindred online community from the same epoch, not limited to university campuses, was found on Reddit in the (now removed) community 'CreepShots', wherein users posted candid photographs of women without their consent.[159] The ensuing discussion followed the same format. These are just two examples of how social media can compound women's nervousness about being seen, and hence evaluated, by others. That is, given that being in the public domain *already* entails scathing evaluations of *every aspect* of a woman's identity, social media pages such as those described above intensify this fear by immortalising and proliferating the scrutiny that fuels it. With this in mind, I am sure I am not alone in understanding Phoebe's fear of leaving her home.

This aspect of Phoebe's account undeniably resonates with the diagnosis 'Agoraphobia', which the *DSM-5* reports to be commonly 'co-morbid' with SAD.[160] It distinguishes between the two thus: 'Agoraphobia should be differentiated from social anxiety disorder based primarily on the situational clusters that trigger fear, anxiety, or avoidance and the cognitive ideation. In social anxiety disorder, the focus is on fear of being negatively evaluated.'[161] Concordant with the first researchers to categorise SAD, Isaac M. Marks and Michael Graham Gelder, I posit that where SAD ends and Agoraphobia begins seems 'rather arbitrary'.[162] Phoebe is a case in point, for her fear of seeing people, or being seen *by* people—and the evaluation that ensues—*causes* her to fear leaving her home to enter public spaces. As before, I am not advocating for a revision of diagnostic criteria, but rather drawing attention to there being 'no very clear line of demarcation'[163] between these diagnoses. This indicates a fundamental flaw with the *DSM-5*'s tenet that these diagnoses are separate, biologically rooted pathologies. By contrast, listening to the accounts of women like Phoebe—and exploring social contributors to their mental distress—can both render their experiences understandable and problematise the notion that they are 'mental illnesses'.

As Phoebe shared her experiences of being seen or watched, another element common to participants' accounts was that women *as a group* are surveyed. Farah told me that 'women are watched' and Phoebe spoke about 'the pressures of gender and like femininity, feeling like you're being watched, feeling like people are talking about your body'. In interviewing participants, it was clear that they understood that women are not merely watched by men but learn to watch each another and, in turn, evaluate one another. Daniella explained: '[Y]ou know women are very judgy of each other? Especially in a group [...] So you always have the thing, "Oh, other people are judging me."'

The pull of this culture of judgement was evident when Daniella told me that, while she believed that 'women care more about what other people think', she herself does not *want* to care, but is unable to shake this concern completely: 'I really don't care, but [...] subconsciously, I do, and it's really annoying.' In addition to judgement, both Daniella and Phoebe alluded to a culture of competition among women which, per McRobbie's reading of Foucault, 'is a defining feature of the rise of neoliberal society':[164]

> Phoebe: [W]hen I went to university [...] I'd always like look at my smaller friends and be really jealous.
>
> Daniella: [Women] seem to always be in competition with each other [...] They're always the topic of conversation of each other. And [...] object of scrutiny of each other.

Daniella then put forth that, owing to this culture of judgement and competition, social anxiety is not something a woman either experiences or does not experience, for 'even in the most, you know, confident woman, it's still a source of a bit of anxiety [...] if a woman has social anxiety, I think that's a big part of it. Because it is for me.' Orbach writes on something analogous in her theorising of women's Anorexia, wherein she contends that 'there is a painful continuity between most women's daily experience and that of the anorectic woman. Nearly all women feel the necessity to restrain their appetites and diminish their size'.[165] Ellen and Phoebe made points akin to Daniella's, and indeed Orbach's, in positing that their feelings of unease likely extend to most women:

> Ellen: [M]y cause of social anxiety is that [...] I do not look like what the ideal, sexy, pretty, beautiful woman would look like. And then I'm just paranoid that people are looking at me, thinking, 'Tall,' or whatever [...] I would imagine it's similar for other women.

> Phoebe: I think a lot of my anxiety stems from kind of restrictive understandings of what femininity should be, and how that's like impacted me. I think a lot of women would probably say that as well.

Following this, if *most* women experience *some* social anxiety, owing to being pitched against one another and incessantly evaluated in light of restrictive models of femininity, we return to the question of whether this unease is best framed as a 'mental disorder'.

As Daniella and Phoebe remarked on competition and judgement between women, Phoebe made another, connected point: 'I think that we internalise so much misogyny […] in social occasions because *you feel watched and then you watch yourself*.'[166] Phoebe's words call to mind the thoughts of Sue in discussing women's objectification and resulting self-objectification. He explains that

> The more women report being gazed at, encountering remarks about their appearance, garnering unwanted sexual attention, and experiencing sexual harassment, the more they also objectified themselves and other women as separate sexual beings.[167] Thus women, who are evaluated in an objectified culture regarding physical appearance, come to evaluate their own worthiness or self-esteem based upon appearance and physical attributes. Self-objectification has been found to be negatively related to mental health, happiness, and subjective well-being.[168]

A key point that I wish to draw out of both Sue's exposition and Phoebe's testimony is that women's being watched and objectified leads to their watching and objectifying one other. In turn, they come to *watch and objectify themselves*. How these experiences play out, and how they interact with social anxiety, will be unpacked in the next chapter.

Notes

1. Kathy Deliovsky, 'Normative White Femininity: Race, Gender and the Politics of Beauty', *Atlantis: Critical Studies in Gender, Culture and Social Justice*, 33.1 (2008), 49–59 https://journals.msvu.ca/index.php/atlantis/article/view/429 [accessed 30 January 2023] p. 50.
2. Raewyn Connell, *Gender and Power: Society, the Person, and Sexual Politics* (Stanford, CA: Stanford University Press, 1987), p. 187.
3. Patricia Hill Collins, *Black Sexual Politics: African Americans, Gender, and the New Racism* (New York: Routledge, 2004).

4. Laura T. Hamilton, Elizabeth A. Armstrong, J. Lotus Seeley, and Elizabeth M. Armstrong, 'Hegemonic Femininities and Intersectional Domination', *Sociological Theory*, 37.4 (2019), 315–41 https://doi.org/10.1177/0735275119888248 p. 322. Italics in original.
5. Meeta Jha, *The Global Beauty Industry: Colorism, Racism, and the National Body* (Oxon and New York: Routledge, 2016), p. iii.
6. Deliovsky, 'Normative White Femininity', p. 50.
7. Collins, *Black Sexual Politics*, p. 194.
8. Deliovsky, 'Normative White Femininity', p. 50.
9. Jha, *The Global Beauty Industry*, p. 1.
10. Hamilton et al., 'Hegemonic Femininities', p. 334.
11. 'Lady' *Merriam-Webster Dictionary* (n.d.) https://www.merriam-webster.com/dictionary/lady [accessed 2 February 2023].
12. Elizabeth A. Armstrong, Laura T. Hamilton, Elizabeth M. Armstrong, and J. Lotus Seeley, '"Good Girls": Gender, Social Class, and Slut Discourse on Campus', *Social Psychology Quarterly*, 77.2 (2014), 100–22 https://doi.org/10.1177/01902725145212
    Julie Bettie, *Women without Class: Girls, Race, and Identity* (Berkeley: University of California Press, 2003).
    All cited in Hamilton et al., 'Hegemonic Femininities', p. 328. My emphasis.
13. Valerie Steeves, '"Pretty and Just a Little Bit Sexy, I Guess": Publicity, Privacy, and the Pressure To Perform "Appropriate" Femininity on Social Media', in *EGirls, ECitizens: Putting Technology, Theory and Policy into Dialogue with Girls' and Young Women's Voices*, ed. by Valerie Steeves and Jane Bailey (Ottawa, Ontario: University of Ottawa Press, 2015), 153–73, p. 158.
14. Ibid., p. 163.
15. Joan C. Chrisler and Ingrid Johnston-Robledo, 'Woman's Embodied Self: An Introduction', in *Woman's Embodied Self: Feminist Perspectives on Identity and Image*, ed. by J. C. Chrisler and I. Johnston-Robledo (Washington, DC: American Psychological Association, 2018), 3–14, p. 11.
16. Chimamanda Ngozi Adichie, *We Should All Be Feminists* (London: Fourth Estate, 2014), p. 27.
17. Steeves, '"Pretty and Just a Little Bit Sexy, I Guess"', p. 163.
18. Ibid., p. 161.
19. Ibid., p. 159.
20. Tressie McMillan Cottom, *Thick and Other Essays* (New York: The New Press, 2019), cited in Hamilton et al., 'Hegemonic Femininities', p. 324.
21. Deliovsky, 'Normative White Femininity', p. 50. My emphasis.
22. Steeves, '"Pretty and Just a Little Bit Sexy, I Guess"', p. 159.

23. Akane Kanai, 'Thinking beyond the Internet as a Tool: Girls' Online Spaces as Postfeminist Structures of Surveillance', in Steeves and Bailey, *EGirls, ECitizens*, 83–108, cited in Steeves, '"Pretty and Just a Little Bit Sexy"', p. 170.
24. Meenakshi Gigi Durham, 'Articulating Adolescent Girls' Resistance to Patriarchal Discourse in Popular Media', *Women's Studies in Communication*, 22.2 (1999), 210–29 https://doi.org/10.1080/07491409.1999.10162421 p. 222, cited in Steeves, '"Pretty and Just a Little Bit Sexy, I Guess"', p. 169.
25. Chrisler and Johnston-Robledo, 'Woman's Embodied Self', p. 5.
26. John Berger, *Ways of Seeing* (Harmondsworth: Penguin, 2008), pp. 40–41.
27. Orbach, *Fat Is a Feminist Issue*, p. 30.
28. Deborah L. Rhode, *The Beauty Bias: The Injustice of Appearance in Life and Law* (Oxford: Oxford University Press, 2010), pp. 6–7. My emphasis.
29. Jha, *The Global Beauty Industry*', pp. 3–4.
30. Susie Orbach, *Hunger Strike: Starving amidst Plenty* (London and New York: Karnac, 2005).
31. American Psychiatric Association, *Diagnostic and Statistical Manual of Mental Disorders* [*DSM-5*] (Washington, DC: American Psychiatric Association Publishing, 2013) https://ebookcentral.proquest.com/lib/bham/reader.action?docID=1811753 [accessed 6 January 2021] p. 203.
32. Sandra Lee Bartky, 'Foucault, Femininity, and the Modernization of Patriarchal Power', in *The Politics of Women's Bodies: Sexuality, Appearance, and Behavior*, ed. by Rose Weitz (New York and Oxford: Oxford University Press, 1998), 25–45, pp. 38–39.
33. Ibid.
34. Chrisler and Johnston-Robledo, 'Woman's Embodied Self', p. 12.
35. Bartky, 'Foucault, Femininity, and the Modernization of Patriarchal Power', pp. 33–34.
36. Ibid., p. 34.
37. Ibid., pp. 38–39.
38. E.g. Alexander Szalai (ed.), *The Use of Time: Daily Activities of Urban and Suburban Populations in Twelve Countries* (The Hague: Mouton, 1972).
39. Arlie Hochschild, *The Second Shift: Working Families and the Revolution at Home* (New York: Penguin Books, 2012), p. 3.
40. Ibid.
41. Ibid., pp. 3–4.
42. Naomi Wolf, *The Beauty Myth: How Images of Beauty Are Used against Women* (London: Vintage Books, 1991).
43. Hochschild, *The Second Shift*, p. 9.

44. Ibid.
45. Wendy Chapkis, *Beauty Secrets: Women and the Politics of Appearance* (Boston, MA: South End Press, 1986), cited in Chrisler and Johnston-Robledo, 'Woman's Embodied Self', p. 11.
46. Michel Foucault, *Discipline and Punish* [*Surveiller et Punir*] trans. Alan Sheridan (Harmondsworth: Penguin, 1991[1975]), p. 135.
47. Ibid., p. 136.
48. Ibid.
49. Bartky, 'Foucault, Femininity, and the Modernization of Patriarchal Power'.
50. Ibid., p. 28.
51. Ibid., p. 35.
52. Frances Bozsik, Brooke L. Whisenhunt, Danae L. Hudson, Brooke Bennett, and Jennifer D. Lundgren, '"Thin Is in? Think Again: The Rising Importance of Muscularity in the Thin Ideal Female Body', *Sex Roles*, 79.9–10 (2018), 609–15 https://doi.org/10.1007/s11199-017-0886-0
53. Emily T. Troscianko, *Anorexia and Today's World: Does Modern Society Foster Anorexia?* (2020) https://www.psychologytoday.com/gb/blog/hunger-artist/201008/anorexia-and-todays-world [accessed 24 May 2023].
54. Roberta Sassatelli, 'Fitness Culture', *The Blackwell Encyclopedia of Sociology* (2007), 1–3 https://doi.org/10.1002/9781405165518.wbeosf083.pub2
55. Chrisler and Johnston-Robledo, 'Woman's Embodied Self', p. 13.
56. Ibid.
57. Ibid.
58. Steeves, '"Pretty and Just a Little Bit Sexy, I Guess"', pp. 166–67.
59. Pearl Gabel, 'Plus-size Model Tess Holliday Busts out of Stereotype', *Daily News* (2015) http://www.nydailynews.com/life-style/plus-size-model-tess-holliday-busts-stereotype-article-1.2090500 [accessed 1 February 2015].
60. Tess Holliday, *EffYourBeautyStandards* (n.d.) https://www.instagram.com/effyourbeautystandards/?hl=en [accessed 26 September 2020].
61. Ngaire Donaghue and Anne Clemitshaw, '"I'm Totally Smart and a Feminist… And yet I Want To Be a Waif": Exploring Ambivalence towards the Thin Ideal within the Fat Acceptance Movement', *Women's Studies International Forum*, 35.6 (2012) https://doi.org/10.1016/j.wsif.2012.07.005 p. 415.
62. Bartky, 'Foucault, Femininity, and the Modernization of Patriarchal Power', p. 28.
63. Ibid., p. 38.
64. Ibid.

65. Iris Marion Young, 'Throwing like a Girl: A Phenomenology of Feminine Body Comportment Motility and Spatiality', *Human Studies*, 3.1 (1980), 137–56 https://doi.org/10.1007/BF02331805 cited in Bartky, 'Foucault, Femininity, and the Modernization of Patriarchal Power', p. 36.
66. Marianne Wex, *Let's Take Back Our Space: Female and Male Body Language as a Result of Patriarchal Structures* (Germany: Frauenliteratur Verlag Hermine Fees, 1979), cited in Bartky, 'Foucault, Femininity, and the Modernization of Patriarchal Power', p. 30.
67. Lily Myers, *Shrinking Women* (n.d.) https://genius.com/Lily-myers-shrinking-women-annotated [accessed 26 September 2020].
68. Wex, *Let's Take Back Our Space*, cited in Bartky, 'Foucault, Femininity, and the Modernization of Patriarchal Power', p. 30.
69. For countless examples, see Laura Bates, *Everyday Sexism Project* (n.d.) https://everydaysexism.com/ [accessed 26 September 2021].
70. Thomas Johansson, 'Gendered Spaces: The Gym Culture and the Construction of Gender', *Young*, 4.3 (1996), 32–47 https://doi.org/10.1177/110330889600400303 p. 32.
71. Ibid.
72. Ibid., p. 35.
73. Sue, *Microaggressions*, p. 16.
74. Ibid.
75. Brigid Francis-Devine and Doug Pyper, *The Gender Pay Gap, House of Commons Library Briefing Paper Number 7068* (2020) https://commonslibrary.parliament.uk/research-briefings/sn07068/ [accessed 18 March 2021].
76. Rape Crisis, *About Sexual Violence* (2020) https://rapecrisis.org.uk/get-informed/about-sexual-violence/statistics-sexual-violence/ [accessed 26 September 2020].
77. Gloria Anzaldúa, *Borderlands La Frontera: The New Mestiza* (San Francisco, CA: Aunt Lute Books, 1987), p. 38.
78. Ariane Prohaska and Jeannine A. Gailey, 'Theorizing Fat Oppression: Intersectional Approaches and Methodological Innovations', *Fat Studies*, 8.1 (2019), 1–9 https://doi.org/10.1080/21604851.2019.1534469 p. 1.
79. Helen Hester and Caroline Walters, '"Riots Not Diets!" Sex, Fat Studies, and DIY Activism', *in Fat Sex: New Directions in Theory and Activism*, ed. by Helen Hester and Caroline Walters (Routledge: Oxon and New York, 2016), 17–28, p. 17.
80. Michael S. Kavic, 'Obesity – An "Acceptable" Prejudice', *Journal of the Society of Laparoendoscopic Surgeons*, 5.3 (2001), 201–02 https://www.ncbi.nlm.nih.gov/pmc/articles/PMC3015454/ [accessed 26 September 2020].

81. Kathrine D. Gapinski, Marlene B. Schwartz, and Kelly D. Brownell, 'Can Television Change Anti-fat Attitudes and Behavior?' *Journal of Applied Biobehavioral Research*, 11.1 (2006), 1–28 https://doi.org/10.1111/j.1751-9861.2006.tb00017.x
    J. Fikkan and E. Rothblum, 'Weight Bias in Employment', in *Weight Bias: Nature, Consequences, and Remedies*, ed. by K. D. Brownell, R. M. Puhl, M. B. Schwartz, and L. Rudd (New York, NY: Guilford Publications, 2005), 15–28.
    All cited in Prohaska and Gailey, 'Theorizing Fat Oppression', p. 4.
82. Susan M. Himes and J. Kevin Thompson, 'Fat Stigmatization in Television Shows and Movies: A Content Analysis', *Obesity*, 15.3 (2007), 712–18 https://doi.org/10.1038/oby.2007.635
    Mallory Hussin, Savannah Frazier, and J. Kevin Thompson, 'Fat Stigmatization on YouTube: A Content Analysis', *Body Image*, 8.1 (2011), 90–92 https://doi.org/10.1016/j.bodyim.2010.10.003
    K. Mendoza, 'Seeing through the Layers: Fat Suits and Thin Bodies in *The Nutty Professor* and *Shallow Hal*', in *The Fat Studies Reader*, ed. by E. Rothblum and S. Solovay (New York, NY: NYU Press, 2009), 280–88.
    Katherine Sender and Margaret Sullivan, 'Epidemics of Will, Failures of Self-esteem: Responding to Fat Bodies in the *Biggest Loser* and *What Not To Wear*', *Continuum,* 22.4 (2008), 573–84 https://doi.org/10.1080/10304310802190046
    All cited in Prohaska and Gailey, 'Theorizing Fat Oppression: Intersectional Approaches and Methodological Innovations', *Fat Studies*, 8.1 (2019), 1–9 https://doi.org/10.1080/21604851.2019.1534469 p. 4.
83. Valena Elizabeth Beety, 'Criminality and Corpulence: Weight Bias in the Courtroom', *Seattle Journal for Social Justice*, 11.2 (2013), 523–53 https://digitalcommons.law.seattleu.edu/sjsj/vol11/iss2/4 [accessed 8 February 2023] cited in Prohaska and Gailey, 'Theorizing Fat Oppression', p. 4.
84. Prohaska and Gailey, 'Theorizing Fat Oppression', p. 4.
85. Eunice Y. Chen and Molly Brown, 'Obesity Stigma in Sexual Relationships', *Obesity Research*, 13.8 (2005), 1393–97 https://doi.org/10.1038/oby.2005.168
    Jeannine A. Gailey, 'Fat Shame to Fat Pride: Fat Women's Sexual and Dating Experiences', *Fat Studies*, 1.1 (2012), 114–27 https://doi.org/10.1080/21604851.2012.631113
    D. Gimlin, *Body Work: Beauty and Self-Image in American Culture* (Berkeley: University of California Press, 2002).
    Viren Swami, Laura Steadman, and Martin J. Tovée, 'A Comparison of Body Size Ideals, Body Dissatisfaction, and Media Influence between Female Track Athletes, Martial Artists, and Non-athletes', *Psychology of*

Sport and Exercise, 10.6 (2009), 609–14 https://doi.org/10.1016/j.psychsport.2009.03.003
All cited in Prohaska and Gailey, 'Theorizing Fat Oppression', p. 5.

86. S. B. Bergman, 'Part-time Fatso', in *The Fat Studies Reader*, ed. by E. Rothblum and S. Solovan (New York: New York University Press, 2009), 139–42, cited in Noortje van Amsterdam, 'Big Fat Inequalities, Thin Privilege: An Intersectional Perspective on "Body Size"', *European Journal of Women's Studies*, 20.2 (2013), 155–69 https://doi.org/10.1177/1350506812456461 p. 5.
87. Lee F. Monaghan, 'Big Handsome Men, Bears and Others: Virtual Construction of "Fat Male Embodiment"', *Body & Society*, 11.1 (2005), 81–111 https://doi.org/10.1177/1357034X05052463
Lee F. Monaghan, 'Body Mass Index, Masculinities and Moral Worth: Men's Critical Understandings of "Appropriate" Weight-for-height', *Sociology of Health and Illness*, 29.4 (2007), 584–609 https://doi.org/10.1111/j.1467-9566.2007.01007.x
All cited in van Amsterdam, 'Big Fat Inequalities', p. 5.
88. Victoria Welsby, *About the BBC Show 'Who Are You Calling Fat?'* (2019) http://fiercefatty.com/blog/about-the-bbc-show-who-are-you-calling-fat [accessed 26 September 2020].
89. Deborah Carr and Michael A. Friedman, 'Is Obesity Stigmatizing? Body Weight, Perceived Discrimination, and Psychological Well-being in the United States', *Journal of Health and Social Behavior*, 46.3 (2005), 244–59 https://doi.org/10.1177/002214650504600303
Kirsten K. Davison, Dorothy L. Schmalz, Laurie M. Young, and Leann L. Birch, 'Overweight Girls Who Internalize Fat Stereotypes Report Low Psychological Well-being', *Obesity*, 16.2 (2008), 30–38 https://doi.org/10.1038/oby.2008.451
Carol T. Miller and Kathryn T. Downey, 'A Meta-analysis of Heavyweight and Self-esteem', *Personality and Social Psychology Review*, 3.1 (1999), 68–84 https://doi.org/10.1207/s15327957pspr0301_4
Jennifer A. O'Dea, 'Self-concept, Self-esteem and Body Weight in Adolescent Females: A Three Year Longitudinal Study', *Journal of Health Psychology*, 11.4 (2006), 599–611 https://doi.org/10.1177/1359105306065020
All cited in Prohaska and Gailey, 'Theorizing Fat Oppression', p. 5.
90. S. Solovay and E. Rothblum, 'Introduction', in *The Fat Studies Reader*, ed. by S. Solovay and E. Rothblum, 1–10, cited in van Amsterdam, 'Big Fat Inequalities', *European Journal of Women's Studies*, 20.2 (2013), 155–69 https://doi.org/10.1177/1350506812456461 p. 4.
91. Orbach, *Hunger Strike*, p. 68.

92. Deaux and Greenwood's tenet is most applicable when the norms of the host country and the country of origin are especially disparate. Although Daniella is a white immigrant from a Western European country who emigrated to the UK, Deaux and Greenwood's work can still be useful in theorising her experience.
93. F. Henry and C. Tator, *The Color of Democracy: Racism in Canadian Society* (Toronto: Thompson/Nelson Press, 2009).
J. Zine, 'Unveiled Sentiments: Gendered Islamophobia and Experiences of Veiling among Muslim Girls in a Canadian Islamic School', *Equality and Excellence in Education*, 39.3 (2006), 239–52 https://doi.org/10.1080/10665680600788503
All cited in Kay Deaux and Ronni Michelle Greenwood, 'Crossing Borders: Intersectional Excursions into Gender and Immigration', in *The SAGE Handbook of Gender and Psychology*, ed. by M. K. Ryan and N. R. Branscombepp (London: Sage Publications, 2013), 234–50, p. 241.
94. Deaux and Greenwood, 'Crossing Borders', p. 238.
95. Orbach, *Hunger Strike.*
96. Bartky, 'Foucault, Femininity, and the Modernization of Patriarchal Power', p. 36.
97. Rhode, *The Beauty Bias*, pp. 6–7. My emphasis.
98. Jha, *The Global Beauty Industry*, pp. 3–4.
99. Orbach, *Fat Is a Feminist Issue*, p. 20. My emphasis.
100. Bartky, 'Foucault, Femininity, and the Modernization of Patriarchal Power', p. 36.
101. Ibid.
102. As I explored in Chap. 3, Phoebe believed herself to be autistic. It is noteworthy that eating problems, especially the diagnosis Anorexia Nervosa, have been linked to autism in women. As full discussion of this interplay is beyond the scope of this book, I refer interested readers to Janina Brede, Charli Babb, Catherine Jones, Mair Elliott, Cathy Zanker, Kate Tchanturia, Lucy Serpell, John Fox, and Will Mandy, '"For Me, the Anorexia Is just a Symptom, and the Cause Is the Autism": Investigating Restrictive Eating Disorders in Autistic Women', *Journal of Autism and Developmental Disorders*, 50 (2020), 4280–96 https://doi.org/10.1007/s10803-020-04479-3
103. NHS, *Symptoms: Anorexia Nervosa* (2018) https://www.nhs.uk/conditions/anorexia/symptoms/ [accessed 26 September 2020].
104. APA, *DSM-5*, p. 339.
105. Janet Polivy and Peter C. Herman, 'Diagnosis and Treatment of Normal Eating', *Journal of Consulting and Clinical Psychology*, 55.5 (1987), 635–44 https://doi.org/10.1037/0022-006X.55.5.635 cited in Malson, *The Thin Woman*, p. 90.

106. Chloë Taylor, 'Female Sexual Dysfunction, Feminist Sexology, and the Psychiatry of the Normal', *Feminist Studies*, 41.2 (2015), 259–92 https://doi.org/10.15767/feministstudies.41.2.259 p. 286.
107. APA, *DSM-5*, p. 339.
108. Adi Robertson, 'Reddit Bans "Fat People Hate" and other Subreddits under New Harassment Rules', *The Verge* (2015) https://www.theverge.com/2015/6/10/8761763/reddit-harassment-ban-fat-people-hate-subreddit [accessed 7 January 2021].
109. Lenore F. Monello and Jean Mayer, 'Obese Adolescent Girls: An Unrecognised "Minority" Group?', *American Journal of Clinical Nutrition*, 13.1 (1963), 35–39 https://doi.org/10.1093/ajcn/13.1.35
110. Kathleen LeBesco, *Revolting Bodies? The Struggle To Redefine Fat Identity* (Boston: University of Massachusetts Press, 2004), p. 59.
111. Marilyn Lawrence, *The Anorexic Experience* (London: The Women's Press Ltd., 1984), p. 39.
112. Marilyn Lawrence, 'Anorexia Nervosa – The Control Paradox', *Women's Studies International Quarterly*, 2.1 (1979), 93–101 https://doi.org/10.1016/S0148-0685(79)93118-X p. 93.
113. Ibid., p. 99.
114. Lawrence, 'Anorexia Nervosa', p. 100.
115. MacSween, *Anorexic Bodies*, p. 4.
116. Lawrence, *The Anorexic Experience*, pp. 18–19.
117. Lawrence, 'Anorexia Nervosa', p. 95.
118. Ibid.
119. Ibid., p. 96.
120. APA, *DSM-5*, p. 344.
121. Richard I. Steim and Carol J. Nemeroff, 'Moral Overtones of Food: Judgments of Others Based on What They Eat', *Personality and Social Psychology Bulletin*, 21.5 (1995), 480–90 https://doi.org/10.1177/0146167295215006
122. Ga-Eun Grace Oh and Young Eun Huh, 'Judge Me for What I Eat: Women Choose Low-calorie Labeled Food To Signal Competence', *14th Association for Consumer Research: Gender, Marketing and Consumer Behavior Conference*, 10–11 October 2018, Hilton Anatole, Dallas, Texas, USA.
123. Peter Conrad, 'Wellness as Virtue: Morality and the Pursuit of Health', *Culture, Medicine and Psychiatry*, 18.3 (1994), 385–401 https://doi.org/10.1007/BF01379232
124. Chrisler and Johnston-Robledo, 'Woman's Embodied Self', p. 13.
125. Wolf, *The Beauty Myth*, pp. 193–94.
126. Cecilia Bergh Rosen, 'An Explorative Study of Bulimia and Other Excessive Behaviours', King Gustav V Research Institutue, Karolinska

Institutute, Stockholm, and the Department of Sociology and the School of Social Work, University of Stockholm, Sweden (1988), p. 77.
Daniota Czyzewski and Melanie A. Suhz (eds). *Hilde Bruch, Conversations with Anorexics* (New York: Basic Books, 1988).
David M. Garner, Paul E. Garfinkel, Donald Schwartz, and Michael Thompson, 'Cultural Expectations of Thinness in Women', *Psychological Reports*, 47.2 (1980), 483–91 https://doi.org/10.2466/pr0.1980.47.2.483
Ilana Attie and J. Brooks-Gunn, 'Weight Concerns as Chronic Stressors in Women', in *Gender and Stress*, ed. by Rosalind Barnett, Lois Biener, Rosalind C. Barnett, and Grace K. Baruch (New York: Free Press, 1987), 218–54.
All cited in Wolf, *The Beauty Myth*, p. 195.

127. For a full description of the study, see Ancel Keys, J. Brožek, A. Henschel, O. Mickelsen, and H. L. Taylor, *The Biology of Human Starvation* (2 Vols.) (Minneapolis, Minnesota: University of Minnesota Press, 1950).
128. Todd Tucker, *The Great Starvation Experiment: Ancel Keys and the Men Who Starved for Science* (New York: Free Press, 2006).
129. Orbach, *Bodies*, p. 150.
130. Ibid., p. 6.
131. Lawrence, *The Anorexic Experience*, p. 18.
132. Helen Fielding, *Bridget Jones's Diary* (London: Picador, 1997).
133. Gill, 'Postfeminist Media Culture', p. 150.
134. Ibid., p. 155.
135. Ibid., p. 156.
136. Brumberg, *The Body Project*, cited in Chrisler and Johnston-Robledo, 'Woman's Embodied Self', p. 5.
137. Peter Öberg and Lars Tornstam, 'Body Images among Men and Women of Different Ages', *Ageing and Society*, 19.5 (1999), 629–44 https://doi.org/10.1017/S0144686X99007394 p. 631, cited in Chrisler and Johnston-Robledo, 'Woman's Embodied Self', p. 5.
138. Motivation_Mondays, *I'm Working on Myself, for Myself, by Myself* (2020) https://www.instagram.com/p/CAIrN9MhKqf/ [accessed 27 September 2020].
139. 6amsuccess, *Your Biggest Opponent Is Yourself* (2020) https://www.instagram.com/p/CAXGbi7jsFI/ [accessed 27 September 2020].
140. Harris, *Future Girl*, p. 16.
141. Susan Hopkins, 'The Art of "Girl Power": Femininity, Feminism and Youth Culture in the 1990s', in *Australian Youth Subcultures: On the Margins and in the Mainstream*, ed. by Rob White (Hobart: Australian Clearinghouse for Youth Studies, 1999), p. 95, cited in Harris, *Future Girl*, p. 17.

142. Harris, *Future Girl*, p. 18.
143. Shani Orgad, *Heading Home: Motherhood, Work, and the Failed Promise of Equality* (New York; Chichester, West Sussex: Columbia University Press, 2019), p. 43.
144. Gill, 'Postfeminist Media Culture', p. 153.
145. Ibid.
146. Ibid., cited in Maria Adamson, 'Postfeminism, Neoliberalism and a "Successfully" Balanced Femininity in Celebrity CEO Autobiographies', *Gender, Work and Organization*, 24.3 (2017), 314–27 https://doi.org/10.1111/gwao.12167 p. 317.
147. Gill, 'Postfeminist Media Culture', p. 153.
148. Ibid.
149. Angela McRobbie, 'Notes on the Perfect: Competitive Femininity in Neoliberal Times', *Australian Feminist Studies*, 30.83 (2015), 3–20 https://doi.org/10.1080/08164649.2015.1011485 p. 6.
150. Malson, *The Thin Woman*, p. 155.
151. Ibid.
152. Ibid.
153. Donaghue and Clemitshaw, '"I'm Totally Smart and a Feminist…"', p. 415.
154. Ibid.
155. Chrisler and Johnston-Robledo, 'Woman's Embodied Self', p. 8.
156. Hannah Seligson, 'The Rise of Bodysnarking', *Wall Street Journal*, 16 May 2008, cited in Orbach, *Bodies*, p. 7.
157. These were most popular on university campuses between 2013 and 2014—the time around which they began to be subject to backlash and critique. Although their popularity has since waned, they still exist.
158. Laura Bates, 'Facebook's "Spotted" Pages: Everyday Sexism in Universities for All To See', *The Guardian* (2014) https://www.theguardian.com/lifeandstyle/womens-blog/2014/jan/31/facebooks-spotted-pages-everyday-sexism-universities [accessed 29 July 2020].
159. Andrea Waling, *Explainer: What Are 'Creepshots' and What Can We Do about Them?* (2017) https://theconversation.com/explainer-what-are-creepshots-and-what-can-we-do-about-them-80807 [accessed 30 July 2020].

     Justin Gray, 'Teacher Allegedly Posts Pictures of Students on "CreepShot" Website', *FOX 5 Atlanta* (2012) https://web.archive.org/web/20130601231618/http://www.myfoxatlanta.com/story/19650823/teacher-allegedly-posts-pictures-of-students-on-site [accessed 30 July 2020].
160. APA, *DSM-5*, p. 221.
161. Ibid.
162. Christopher Lane, *Shyness: How Normal Behavior Became a Sickness* (Yale University Press, 2007) https://ebookcentral.proquest.com/lib/bham/reader.action?docID=3420940 [accessed 6 January 2021] pp. 71–72.

163. Eliot Slater and Martin Roth, *Clinical Psychiatry*, 3rd edn (Baltimore: Williams and Wilkins, 1969), pp. 95–96, cited in Lane, *Shyness*, p. 72.
164. McRobbie, 'Notes on the Perfect'.
165. Orbach, *Hunger Strike*, p. 78.
166. My emphasis.
167. Melanie S. Hill and Ann R. Fischer, 'Examining Objectification Theory: Lesbian and Heterosexual Women's Experiences With Sexual- and Self-objectification', *The Counseling Psychologist*, 36.5 (2008), 745–76 https://doi.org/10.1177/0011000007301669
Janet K. Swim, Lauri L. Hyers, Laurie L. Cohen, and Melissa J. Ferguson, 'Everyday Sexism: Evidence for its Incidence, Nature, and Psychological Impact from Three Daily Diary Studies', *Journal of Social issues*, 57.1 (2001), 31–53 https://doi.org/10.1111/0022-4537.00200
168. Barbara L. Fredrickson and Tomi-Ann Roberts, 'Objectification Theory: Toward Understanding Women's Lived Experiences and Mental Health Risks', *Psychology of Women Quarterly*, 21.2 (1997), 173–206 https://doi.org/10.1111/j.1471-6402.1997.tb00108.x cited in Sue, *Microaggressions*, p. 170.

CHAPTER 6

The Ideal Self

In the previous chapter, we saw that women's social anxiety was not only predicated on others' perceptions of their bodies, but that it extended to others' perceptions of their entire selves. In this chapter, I use the work of anti-psychiatrist R. D. Laing to explore how participants experienced this. I examine how they described cultivating an acceptable outward, or 'false', self which comports with feminine norms and others' expectations. This then stands in contradistinction to their 'true' self—who they *really* are and how they *really* feel. I probe how gendered social conditions give rise to this cleavage and, in turn, how many of the women's accounts evoke the idea of an 'inner critic'. In so doing, I find significant overlap between their experiences and the *DSM-5*'s 'Dissociative Disorders'. In the spirit of Laing's work, I put forth that considering women's socialisation renders these experiences intelligible. Moreover, given that this group of diagnostic categories has hitherto not been linked to SAD, I contend that the inner world of the socially anxious woman is vastly under-researched and poorly understood. As such, it warrants greater attention if we are to render this position understandable and have any hope of alleviating her distress.

K. Masters, *Feminist and Anti-Psychiatry Perspectives on 'Social Anxiety Disorder'*,
https://doi.org/10.1007/978-3-031-48707-1_6

Watching the Self

I invite the reader to recall Phoebe's words at the end of the last chapter: '[Y]ou feel watched and then *you watch yourself*.'[1] Phoebe's comment is reminiscent of ideas in Michel Foucault's *Discipline and Punish*.[2] In brief, Foucault uses philosopher Jeremy Bentham's Panopticon to explore self-surveillance. In this 'perfect prison', since only the central observation point therein, and not what or who is inside, is visible from the cells, the inmates do not know whether they are being observed at any given time. Inmates thus *behave as though they are being observed, irrespective of whether they are or not.* Consequently, they effectively watch themselves, or engage in self-surveillance and, by extension, self-regulation. They have internalised the 'inspecting' gaze of the surveyor.[3] Art critic John Berger provides insight into the relevance of this concept for women. That is, a woman is aware of herself as 'an object of vision',[4] incessantly accompanied by 'her own image of herself':[5] 'Women watch themselves being looked at.'[6] Susie Orbach has also written on this phenomenon, contending that 'women are taught to see themselves from the outside as candidates for men':[7] they 'assum[e] the gaze of the observer'.[8]

In the interests of exploring contemporary manifestations of self-surveillance, I return to Valerie Steeves's work on young women's social media use. Steeves contends that this demographic is 'under a high degree of social pressure to conform to "the norms of femininity" and typically judge themselves through the lens of peer acceptance'.[9] While Berger and Orbach describe women's surveying themselves, Steeves alludes to women's surveying their *online* selves. Thus, their social media accounts are never far from their minds. Ellen mentioned this in describing her teenage cousin: '[S]he is constantly [...] I can see how she lives her life through social media.' Ellen's words echo Berger's tenet that, in everyday life, a woman is accompanied by 'her own image of herself'[10]—or, we might now say, 'her own Instagram profile'. I am sure I am not alone in recalling having been at a party, on holiday, or even at the gym, and witnessing others taking photographs or videos which seem not to be for posterity or to immortalise a cherished memory or special occasion (though these certainly may form part of the motivation). Rather, these photographs and videos appear to serve primarily as fodder for one's social media profiles. Ria had observed this while on holiday:

> [W]e climbed up one of the Mayan pyramids, and at the top, you saw people like getting selfies like on the edge [...] And then the other thing as well [...] we saw this woman: really, really stunning woman in like a bikini [...] she was taking like a selfie and she had like a friend next to her with like a big metal sheet, to get the lighting right [...] And you're like, 'Gosh, that is a thing.'

With the rise in popularity of social media, we can see that women, such as the bikini-clad woman Ria described, increasingly live their daily lives governed by what will look favourable online, as opposed to living in the moment and experiencing the world through their own eyes. Ria encapsulated this when she said, '[T]hat one minute of the day where I might be doing a stretch [...] "Oh gosh, we've got to make you do it in the sunset now" [...] and make sure it makes a good photo.'

Writer Susan Sontag has said that 'the camera makes everyone a tourist in other people's reality, and eventually in one's own'.[11] If we replace 'the camera' with 'social media', we have a descriptor for how platforms such as Instagram foster detachment from first-person experience in our time. Every day, women are accompanied by the questions, 'How am I looking today? How are my knees, my breasts, my buttocks, etc.?'[12] Now, we are increasingly accompanied by the additional question: '[H]ow can I capture what I am doing so that it will look good on my social media profiles?' Ria had trouble resisting the pressure to engage in this practice:

> [I]t really like frustrates me, because I think there's a part of me as well that goes, 'Should I be joining in with that?' You know, like, there's this genuine bit of conflict, and then I'm like, 'No, don't be stupid.'

In discussing women's experiencing the world through their own eyes (or not), the work of anti-psychiatrist R. D. Laing starts to become relevant. One of Laing's case studies, Joan, is quoted as having said to him, 'It was only when I looked at myself through your eyes that I could see anything good.'[13] The notion that women regard themselves with *male* eyes is reminiscent of feminist film theorist Laura Mulvey's term 'the male gaze'. Originally coined to describe the role of the passive female and active male in narrative film, the theory of 'the male gaze' holds that the viewer is assumed to be male, and women are looked at or displayed.[14]

Women may come to internalise the 'male gaze', which brings us to Janet Holland et al.'s research on young people's narratives on heterosexuality. Holland and colleagues propose that young women have a 'male-in-the-head', which comprises 'the surveillance power of [...] male-dominated and institutionalised heterosexuality'.[15] A woman, therefore,

> Through her subordinated participation in his performance she is inducted into the world of heterosexual sexuality, where she has to manage her femininity according to the 'male-in-the-head' or take the consequences of resistance. Under this gaze, her sexual identity, subjectivity and desire are silenced.[16]

Kathy Deliovsky's writings add nuance to Holland et al.'s work, for she contends that women must learn to 'behav[e] appropriately by the rules of normative *white* femininity, which is in line with compulsory *white* heterosexuality'.[17] In turn, women's behaviours come to be shaped by the expectations and interests of others, particularly white heterosexual men. Perhaps this is to what Laing's case study, Joan, is alluding. Indeed, one of Holland et al.'s participants 'comments on a sense of being assessed by someone else's standards'.[18] This gives insight into why women might be concerned with how they are perceived: how they can behave and, ultimately, who they can *be* rests upon others' opinions.

In applying self-surveillance to women, it would be remiss not to consider Sandra Lee Bartky's explicitly feminist reading of Foucault. In particular, Bartky tells us that 'a panoptical male connoisseur resides within the consciousness of most women'[19] and that women learn to look 'at themselves from the outside'.[20] Novelist Margaret Attwood's words paint a similar picture in that she describes 'the ever-present watcher peering through the keyhole [...] in your own head [...] You are a woman with a man inside watching a woman. You are your own voyeur'.[21] In the section that follows, I will deploy these ideas in exploring women's relationship with their bodies and, in turn, their selves.

The Body and the Self

One scholar who has written extensively on how women are socialised to view their bodies is Susie Orbach. In her book on women and Anorexia Nervosa, *Hunger Strike*, she describes how the adolescent girl develops 'a split between her body and her self', since '[h]er body is rapidly being presented to her and being perceived by her as an artifact'.[22] And just as our culture views the body, particularly its thinness, as reflecting one's character, it also requires that a ***woman's*** body 'expresses both her oneness with the culture and her individuality'.[23] For Orbach, a woman's body is therefore 'both divorced from and yet reflective of who [...] she is'.[24] This demand necessitates careful curation which is not without cost: Joan C. Chrisler and Ingrid Johnston-Robledo contend that too great a focus on the body project 'encourages self-objectification, a form of disconnection of body from self'.[25]

As such, women may come to view 'their bodies from the outside, as if they were commodities'.[26] In doing so, a woman 'measures how far from the projected norm she is'.[27] On this norm, Deliovsky notes that '[h]omogenized representations of "whitified" feminine beauty become normalized and function as models against which women continually measure, judge, discipline and correct themselves'.[28] Olivia related this to social anxiety, noting that norms such as these 'encourage girls to feel more cripplingly self-conscious than boys in how they must present themselves'.

Orbach further characterises a woman's perception of her own body as 'visual acuity turned in on itself':[29] a woman comes to view her body 'almost as one removed'.[30] This detachment ran through the young women's testimonies in Holland et al.'s research, since

> [T]hey are under pressure to construct their bodies into a model of femininity which is both inscribed on the surface, through such skills as dress, make-up and dietary regimes, and disembodied, in the sense of detachment from their sensuality and alienation from their material bodies.[31]

These themes all evoke the depersonalisation in what the *DSM-5* calls 'Depersonalization/Derealization Disorder'. This is described as 'clinically significant persistent or recurrent depersonalization (i.e., experiences of unreality or detachment from one's mind, self, or body)'[32] or feeling 'as if one were an outside observer of one's mental processes or body'.[33] Anthropologist Emily Martin writes on these sorts of experiences, reporting 'a fair amount of fragmentation and alienation in women's general conceptions of body and self'.[34] Following Martin, if Anglo-American culture is conducive to women's conceiving of their bodies in this way, the claim that this constitutes a discrete psychiatric disorder,[35] or even a psychiatric disorder at all, should be regarded with suspicion. In the same way that appearance concerns and eating problems are 'on a hazy continuum with the banal',[36] women's experiencing *some* depersonalisation is inevitable given the way that they are socialised to view their bodies.

Depersonalisation such as this bespeaks a specifically feminine Cartesian dualism. Although some participants—explicitly and implicitly—rejected Cartesian dualism, as in Chap. 3, we will soon see that they also sometimes spoke in such a way as to endorse it. This suggests that conceptualising ourselves in this way is so ingrained that it is difficult to rid ourselves of it completely. It also suggests—and this might be exactly *why* it is so ingrained—constraints imposed by the language available for us to speak about ourselves. Laing states that this is the case for how we think of psychiatric patients, since our language 'consists of words which split man up verbally'.[37] Phoebe also hinted at this in telling me that 'our language is kind of imbued with the like disciplining of women'.

One of ways by which the above said dualism manifests, Orbach tells us, is that many women come to view their body as 'an "it" rather than their home'.[38] This was evident when Phoebe recalled: '[M]y body wasn't kind of maybe as thin as it "should" have been.' By extension, Orbach puts forth that we 'judge our appearance through a hyper-critical lens, objectifying our faults'.[39] This was realised in the words of Ellen when she explained how, on losing weight, her breasts 'were really small [and] I was like, "This is great!"' Ellen later focused on another part of her body, telling me, 'I only want a bigger arse [...] my arse is flat as a pancake.' Ellen's latter remark invokes Deliovsky's exposition of how definitions of white normative feminine beauty might appropriate 'racial and ethnic markers, for example full lips or "big butts"', which 'become markers of beauty when on the bodies of white women'.[40] As well as regarding our bodies as collections of markers or things, Orbach argues that women see their bodies, on the whole, as products that 'we manufacture and create'.[41] This parallels Harris's conceptualisation of the body-as-project, and Ellen married this notion with the idea that the body is indeed a collection of things in telling me that her 'Instagram feed is literally, "How to get like the perfect arse at the gym".'

Chrisler and Johnston-Robledo describe these 'body-related self-improvement projects' as women's 'attempt to manage their body image and self-identity'.[42] Orbach speaks to this in her theorising of women's anorexia, which she frames as 'the excruciating spectacle of women actually *transforming* their bodies'.[43] And while Chrisler and Johnston-Robledo tell us that the body project is something undertaken by women in light of '[t]he cultural tendency to define a woman as her body',[44] 'or as her face',[45] the rationale given by Orbach is farther-reaching. That is, *anorexic* women transform their bodies 'to deal with the contradictory requirements of their role in late twentieth-century America and England'.[46] Perhaps, in light of these contradictory requirements, socially anxious women likewise strive to transform their *whole selves*. Orbach goes on to frame anorexia as 'a metaphor of our times – an especially poignant statement of the way that the predicaments of life in late twentieth-century capitalism can be experienced by the individual woman'.[47] Phoebe's account paralleled this when she explained societal contributors to her own, and other women's, social anxiety:

> [W]hen you throw in like fucking capitalism and how that fucks everyone up, but especially women, because it profits off women's anxieties […] in the sense of beauty aesthetics and how that creates anxiety […] [T]he way that gender and capitalism interlink has had a massive impact on me as a person […] it impacts all of us.

Building upon Phoebe's words, one of the particular experiences that impacts us, as women, is self-surveillance. It is here that I would like to revisit a remark made by Ellen in the preceding chapter, where she stated that it is not only women's *bodies* which are surveyed, but that we are 'surveyed on how we behave as well'. Morag MacSween articulates how this surveying is internalised, arguing that 'women watch what they eat, how they dress, talk, sit, walk and behave'.[48] Olivia's account mirrored this when she described how her social anxiety encompasses many aspects of her self-presentation: 'I identify as having SAD in that I feel self-conscious and hyper-conscious of my appearance, body language, mannerisms, what I say and how I sound whenever I'm in a social situation.'

Farah's experience followed this, but it was somewhat distinct from that of participants who were concerned expressly with how their *bodies* were perceived, many of whom also related struggles around eating. Instead, Farah characterised her social anxiety thus: 'It wasn't about […] [t]he image of my body, but it was about the image that generally as a person I have […] intellectually.' Farah's account therefore intimates an analogy of sorts. Social anxiety, like eating problems, may arise in response to a narrow bodily norm. But it may also arise in response to 'raced, classed, and gendered'[49] norms of *behaviour*. As such, while Orbach argues that anorexic women are in 'a struggle to reshape themselves physically and emotionally',[50] socially anxious women seem to be in a struggle to reshape their *entire selves*.

In the interests of unpacking this further, I ask the reader again to recall Ellen's narrative from the preceding chapter, where she described social media's deleterious effect on her body image. Whereas Ellen followed public figures and 'influencer' accounts, and her concerns centred mainly on her body, Ria's social media use was different:

> I'd go online […] looking at where people were, and I still do that, I compare where I am in life to where other people are […] Ooh, so and so's got kids, and, you know, they're doing this and doing this.

While Ellen's social anxiety seems to be precipitated by her being exposed to a bodily norm, Ria's seems to be triggered by her exposure to a norm which is far more encompassing. Through following people she knew, or had known, online, the norm to which she is exposed incorporates other aspects of the self, such as achievements and life advancement.

Ria's testimony also reminds us how social media is intertwisted with women's social anxiety. Social media renders all facets of users' lives visible, with an individual's profile commonly constituting a highlight reel. The viewer compares this to their own life: inevitably, this seems lacklustre. What Ria is describing is akin to 'passive use' of Facebook, where the user observes others' highlight reels, but does not interact with them or engage in content production of their own. One study, while not purporting that passive Facebook use simply *causes* social anxiety, suggests an association between the two.[51] In the same vein, another study reports a correlation between 'Facebook use intensity and social comparison frequency', with the latter also being correlated with 'the frequency of having a negative feeling from comparison'.[52] Social comparison is defined as 'where individuals compare themselves as having more positive (downward comparison) or negative (upward comparison) qualities than others'.[53] Ria's account evoked social comparison insofar as she reported often thinking, '[T]here's where I am, that's where they are', on viewing others' profiles.

We might consider this aspect of Ria's testimony through the lens of Laura T. Hamilton and colleagues' exposition of a hierarchy of femininities. That is, '[M]arginalized femininities are those cultural ideals of womanhood that sit just below hegemonic femininities and sometimes even benefit from hegemonic femininities, while subordinated femininities (e.g., those that reflect Blackness and poverty) hold the bottom.'[54] Ria's social comparison could hence be read in terms of her seeking to situate her own femininity, as a British-Punjabi woman, in this hierarchy. It also draws links with the importance of 'belonging' in social anxiety, about which many participants, including Ria, spoke in Chap. 3.

Although Ria's social media use was distinct from Ellen's, their narratives had one thing in common. In much the same way that Ellen seemed aware that her social media use was deleterious to her body image, Ria was conscious that how she used social media 'might feed into social anxiety to some extent'. That is, she reported the following sentiment: 'I've got to look like I'm, you know, managing everything beautifully [...] this person's managing everything beautifully so I should also be doing the same.'

Ria's nod to social media as a vehicle by which we can depict our lives through a rosy lens provides a segue into what Orbach has termed '[t]he postmodern myth of self-invention'.[55] In terms of the body, this is exemplified by the normalisation of cosmetic surgery[56] and, like other forms of beauty work, it is imbued with whiteness. As Deliovsky describes, we have 'Asian wom[e]n [...] getting "double eyelid" surgery, Jewish women getting a "nose job" and African women bleaching their skin'.[57] This 'quest [...] to construct a different body'[58] finds a counterpart in what psychiatrist Peter D. Kramer coins 'cosmetic psychopharmacology':[59] that is, the 'reshaping of personality traits by medication'.[60] Remoulding and remaking, in all their forms, necessitate a woman's watching herself so that, as Berger tells us, '[S]he comes to consider the surveyor and the surveyed within her as the two constituent yet always distinct elements of her identity as a woman.'[61] There is deep resonance between Berger's remarks and anti-psychiatrist Laing's most notable opus, *The Divided Self*,[62] and it is to this that I now turn.

The False Self

The above mentioned work is premised on Laing's case studies of individuals labelled 'schizoid'. One of the defining features of such individuals is that they have two 'personas': a 'real' self, which remains hidden, and a 'false' self, which interacts with the world at large. In a nod to Joan C. Chrisler's finding that 'dualistic discourse'—'Jekyll & Hyde'[63]—featured in PMS self-help books, we might here draw on the words of Dr Henry Jekyll himself: '[Wo]man is not truly one, but truly two.'[64] In *The Divided Self*, Laing posits that psychosis[65] results from the tension between these two selves. In so doing, he seeks to render this experience comprehensible and, in turn, refutes its construal as a medical problem. Although *this* book does not deal with psychosis specifically, I find utility in Laing's conception of selves and I am not the first with interests in feminist approaches to mental distress to do so. Orbach, in theorising women's Anorexia, follows the work of psychoanalyst Donald W. Winnicott whose writings on selves have much in common with Laing's.

Citing Winnicott, Orbach tells us that if, in infancy, the baby girl's needs remain unmet, for instance, 'if [...] she has been left crying',[66] then she thinks that 'it must be because of some action on [...] her part, some failure of [...] hers. It is the baby rather than the care-giver who feels at fault or inadequate'.[67] As a result, '[A] kind of split takes place inside [the baby's] mind. A part of them stays eager and attentive to the mother, while another part is watchful for what it is about themselves that will be received rather than rejected.'[68] As such, the baby, 'in bringing forward parts of [...] herself that suit the mother',[69] develops 'a false self'[70] which is 'more pleasing'[71] and features 'an overdevelopment of certain aspects of the self at the expense of other aspects':[72] the false self comprises the aspects to which the caregiver will respond favourably.[73] The true self, by contrast, 'remains undeveloped'[74] because it has been 'split off and repressed'.[75] Crucially, the false self develops because the baby girl is 'wary of what emanates from [...] herself'.[76] This wariness is undeniably reminiscent of the self-surveillance in which socially anxious women engage due to being concerned with how they are perceived by others.

Now, to delve into the infancies of the women I interviewed for this book would be a difficult, if not impossible, endeavour, and to do so is beyond the book's scope. However, while Laing contends that the first year of life is important, he tells us that childhood and adolescence 'may still have great effect one way or the other'.[77] Extrapolating this, I suggest that girls', and later women's, unrelenting socialisation across the entirety of their lifetimes is conducive to developing a true and false self dyad. To support this, I will examine Laing's tenets on the body and the false self while asking the reader to bear in mind an earlier contention from Orbach: that women come to view their bodies as external objects. On this point, Laing tells us that an individual with a false self 'experiences himself as being more or less divorced or detached from his body [...] the body is felt more as one object among other objects in the world than as the core of the individual's own being'.[78] That is, the body is 'felt as the core of the false self, which a detached, disembodied, "inner", "true" self looks on at with tenderness, amusement, or hatred'.[79] The true self's 'functions come to be observation, control, and criticism'.[80]

While having much in common with the words of Orbach, Laing's description also evokes Dissociative Identity Disorder (DID)—another of the *DSM-5*'s Dissociative Disorders—wherein one becomes a depersonalised observer 'of their "own" speech and actions'.[81] His description is also reminiscent of Depersonalization/Derealisation Disorder, on which I touched earlier, wherein '[t]he depersonalization experience can sometimes be one of a split self, with one part observing and one participating, known as an "out-of-body experience" in its most extreme form'.[82] This depersonalisation is described as an experience of being 'an outside observer with respect to one's thoughts, feelings, sensations, body, or actions'.[83] Considering Orbach's writings on women's bodies; feminist readings of Foucault's self-surveillance; and Berger's exposition of women's being divided into surveyor and surveyed, we can begin to understand why women, especially *socially anxious* women, might have experiences akin to these. Laing tells us that:

> This *identification of the self with the phantasy of the person by whom one is seen* may contribute decisively to the characteristics of the observing self [...] this observing often kills and withers anything that is under scrutiny. The individual now has a persecuting observer in the very core of his being [...] he retains his awareness of himself as an object in the eyes of another by observing himself as the other.[84]

I am reminded here of Amy who, when recounting how she feels socially anxious with her friends, recalled asking herself, '[H]ow do I appear to them?' Laing continues:

> [H]e lends the other his eyes in order that he may continue to be seen; he then becomes an object in his own eyes. But the part of himself who looks into him, has developed the persecutory features he has come to feel the real person outside him to have.[85]

Laing is describing an individual who becomes 'compulsively preoccupied with the sustained observation of his own mental and/or bodily processes':[86] the true self is 'extremely aware of itself, and observes the false self, usually highly critically'.[87]

Orbach's work again has salience for how this plays out in the case of the socially anxious woman. In an effort to create a new self that will be more accepted, Orbach posits that the *anorexic* woman develops a false self.[88] Both Olivia's and Ria's testimonies were in line with this insofar as they described how their socialisation had instilled in them that they, as women, must please others:

> Olivia: [G]irls are socialised to think that being feminine involves being passive and pleasing [...] to be in the company of [...] girls are made to feel like it is in their role to please others and be agreeable [...] So girls/women may learn to just give in to the passivity.
>
> Ria: [T]he idea that you've got to be nice and agreeable [...] you've got to, you know, basically be on-tap for these men [...] In a sense of [...] any Punjabi family gathering.

Yet, these women's socialisation, and how they construct a false self, is shaped not only by their gender but by their race and ethnicity—white women's experience for Olivia; British-Punjabi women's experience for Ria. Olivia's testimony in particular calls to mind Kimberlé Crenshaw's quoting of the maxim that 'men and women are taught to see men as independent, capable, powerful; men and women are taught to see women as dependent, limited in abilities, and passive'.[89] Olivia's remarks further paralleled this adage, since she also said that '[b]oys and girls are socialised to think that being masculine involves being assertive, confident and in control, taking a leadership role, and boys are encouraged to be masculine'. But these aphorisms are largely applicable to white women's experience, with Crenshaw noting that, for example, 'Black men are not viewed as powerful, nor are Black women seen as passive.'[90] As such, taking into account 'the experiential base upon which many feminist insights are grounded'[91]—white women's experience—is important. Doing so can tell us why Olivia's words resonate so strongly with Crenshaw's maxim; Ria's, somewhat less so. It also provides a window into the sociocultural milieux from which each of these women's false selves is born.

What Olivia's and Ria's accounts *do* have in common is their linkage to Chrisler and Johnston-Robledo's observation that women are expected to 'be warm, approachable, giving, yielding, and cater to others' needs before their own'.[92] This calls to mind Virginia Woolf's description of the Victorian 'Angel in the House', who 'never had a mind but preferred to sympathize always with the minds and wishes of others'.[93] In a similar vein, Lisa Downing notes that women are 'supposed [...] to be life-giving, to be nurturing, to be *for the other*, and therefore literally *self-less*'.[94] In turn, women have the experience of never constructing a self that is meaningfully true.

One of the means by which women respond to these expectations is noted by Holland et al., who argue that '[y]oung women […] make a distinction between the presentation of themselves that men respond to'[95]—we might call this their 'false self'—'and what they think of as their "real self"'.[96] According to Orbach, the real self, owing to having its needs unmet, views itself as 'bad': it feels 'the necessity to protect others from its presence'.[97] This necessity, or the need to put others first, harks back to participants' narratives on help-seeking from Chap. 3: many of them only did so to allay others' worries or at their behest. Amy articulated this requirement when explaining how she felt that her 'responsibility […] to make other people comfortable' was something that 'society has really ingrained in me as a woman'. In short, as Downing writes, women are 'supposed […] to be *for the other*'.[98]

Being for the Other

Both Amy's and Downing's remarks speak to Susie Orbach and Luise Eichenbaum's tenet that a woman 'must *defer* to others, follow their lead, articulate her needs only in relation to theirs'.[99] Orbach continues this train of thought in *Hunger Strike*, theorising that a woman's creation of a false self 'is an attempt to take up and meet the projections of others'.[100] Indeed, Laing posits that the false self is contingent on others for its definition.[101] This calls forth the part of Farah's narrative which resonated with those of individuals diagnosed with Selective Mutism. In brief, due to being accompanied by memories of how she had behaved in past situations, Farah felt compelled to behave as others had come to expect. To borrow Orbach's turn of phrase, women learn to 'tune our antennae to adjust to others' expectations'.[102] Ria's testimony also espoused this idea:

> [T]here's a social pressure […] the idea that you want to sort of make your parents proud […] your grandparents proud and have them be able to sort of show off about you […] I'm a bit of an approval so-and-so.

The approval about which Ria speaks is something on which Orbach has also written. The need for this arises from society's insistence that women suppress their *own* needs—or are '*self-less*'[103]—which causes them to 'not feel good within themselves'.[104] Winning others' approval therefore 'temporarily quiets the uneasy feelings inside'.[105] Phoebe shared an early memory of needing approval, telling me, 'I remember [...] some boys in my school, who I was friends with [...] and I kind of wanted them to like me'.

On this point, Orbach discusses a hypothetical woman who, having not been 'encouraged to develop her initiating part and draw a sense of authenticity and strength from that [...] is victimized by a constant need for affirmation from external sources'.[106] While Orbach was writing in 2005, Steeves's research on young women's social media use, published in 2015, represents a contemporary take on this notion. Steeves tells us that the 'peer surveillance' inherent in social media teaches women 'to look for external *male* validation, and the easiest way to attain that validation [is] to conform to gendered stereotypes'.[107] Though she did not explicitly mention *male* validation, the need for *external* validation came to the fore when I was conversing with Ria. Ria explained that she saw this in her sister who 'recently got a promotion [...] She's doing really, really well. But I know with her, she still needs to hear it from other people'. That Ria's sister, who—to my knowledge—does *not* experience social anxiety, requires external validation would suggest that this need is common to a lot of women. Indeed, Ria later pondered, 'Do women need that external validation more and, if so, why?'

When discussing external sources which provide validation, one might initially think only of other *people*. However, Ria revealed how she had found this in other ways during her school and university years:

> In our class, for example, we'd take a test, and the guys would come out, 'It was easy, that was easy.' And then the results would come out and I'd done better than any of them [...] now we don't go by exams [...] so we don't have the reassurance of, 'Oh, it's ok, I'm good' [...] after a while, it's going to be a bit like, 'Ok, maybe [boys/men] are as good as they say they are and I'm not as good.' [...] [W]hat is it [...] maybe not all women [...] what is it that stops people, maybe like us, from sort of accepting that the record states that we're okay, in general? [...] because like once the 'safety mechanism' of external feedback's gone...

The hard numbers by which Ria used to obtain validation might make us think of something inherent to social media: the 'like' function. This reveals, as Steeves tells us, how each photograph that young women post 'is judged by their peers'.[108] The 'like' function therefore represents a quantification of external approval. Just as Ria's test scores used to provide evidence that she was doing well academically, the number of 'likes' on a woman's photograph tells her that she is doing normative femininity well (or not, as the case may be).

Ria's pondering vis-à-vis the need for validation draws links with the thoughts of author and psychoanalyst Marion Milner, who muses that 'this might explain why I was so desperately dependent upon what people thought of me [...] the fact that something had been said made it true'.[109] In this vein, Orbach contends that women's socialisation is conducive to them having a shaky sense of self. They thus come to need reassurance from others, for their very identities, or selves, depend on it. But besides their socialisation, women's precarious sense of self can be traced to another source: gendered conflicts.

The False Self and Conflicts

In *The Divided Self*, anti-psychiatrist Laing proposes that the 'schizoid' individual experiences a split in their self between a hidden, authentic self and an outward persona. It is through reading Laing's work that we can understand not only how conflicts are implicated in this split, but how the gendering of these conflicts is intrinsic to the socially anxious woman's experience. Elaine Showalter has noted that a number of Laing's case studies feature women who are struggling with resolving conflicting ideas about femininity. Yet, '[T]hese potential theories of gender are not developed in themselves.'[110] This section begins to redress this oversight, as many participants reported these sorts of struggles—struggles arising from women's being, to quote Orbach, 'pushed and pulled in opposing directions'.[111] For example, Ellen told me about being a *gourmand* in a climate of self-denial and body shape ideals:

> My Instagram feed is literally, 'How to get like the perfect arse at the gym,' and then the next one down will be like, 'How to make the cheesiest pizza.' I'm like, 'I'm just going to constantly be battling this.'

This sort of clashing appeared in Ellen's narrative earlier on. In Chap. 5, she expressed pro-body-positivity and anti-diet-culture sentiment but struggled to apply these attitudes to herself. The thoughts that Ellen reveals to the world thus seem different from those she holds within. Olivia mentioned a parallel conflict in Chap. 4, where she spoke about a 'girls can do anything' narrative which jars with most girls' socialisation. She explained: 'I struggle being assertive and speaking my mind because it seems contradictory when at the same time I'm always trying to be pleasing and nice and untroublesome and thoughtful of how others might feel.' Being 'pleasing and nice' could be described as Olivia's false self, which society expects her to exhibit, and which she displays to stave off negative evaluation; 'being assertive and speaking my mind' is how she *really* wants to behave. Analogously, Ellen *wants* to be wholeheartedly body positive and anti-diet culture; inevitably, and to her regret, she has internalised some of the fatphobia with which our society is replete.

Both of these women's accounts invoke a phenomenon which Dana Crowley Jack and Diana Dill have termed 'self-silencing'. This is defined as 'the inhibition of thoughts and feelings to avoid relationship conflict and loss'.[112] In discussing self-silencing, they utilise the concept of a 'divided self', that is, 'behaving in a compliant manner to live up to female role imperatives whilst feeling angry inside'.[113] This parallels Laing's divided self—not only in name, but in definition—wherein '[t]he basic split in his being is along the line of cleavage between his outward compliance and his inner withholding of compliance'.[114]

Another example of a divided self can be found in psychoanalyst Joan Riviere's *Womanliness as a Masquerade*. Therein, Riviere opens by observing that the homosexual man might overplay his heterosexuality as a compensatory mechanism.[115] Likewise, women who 'wish for masculinity' employ femininity as a façade with the aim of averting anxiety; concealing traits which are not acceptably feminine; and escaping negative consequences from men.[116] This speaks to Angela McRobbie's thoughts on 'the post-feminist masquerade and the perfect [which] display highly normative and ultimately pleasing femininity where any aggression is entirely inner-directed'.[117] Notions akin to these are also found in Arlie Hochschild's opus *The Managed Heart*. Hochschild proposes that we are oftentimes confronted by a discontinuity between what we feel and what we feel we 'should' feel. We negotiate this disconnect by appealing to 'feeling rules' in terms of what we feel we owe to those around us.[118]

In the interests of building upon Hochschild's thesis, I argue that women are particularly vulnerable to experiencing this disconnect in light of 'the enduring power of the expectation that [they] should *be for others*'.[119] The remarks of Laing's case study, Joan, are once again germane, for she is reported as having said: 'With everyone else I was trying to change myself to please them'.[120] This sentiment is also noted in one of

Susie Scott's shy case studies, Georgia, who, in '"tailoring" herself to fit in with other people [...] found it increasingly difficult to retain a coherent sense of identity and ontological security, feeling as if the different faces of her social self were fragmenting'.[121] Scott then cites another of Laing's case studies, Julie, who 'felt that she was "tailor-made" to meet the demands of others'.[122]

Remaining with Laing's case studies, *The Divided Self* deals with the schizoid's deployment of a false self: a strategy adopted because of not fitting in. The closest contemporary diagnostic category to Laing's 'schizoid' can be found in the *DSM-5*'s 'Schizoid Personality Disorder' (SPD). This is characterised by a preference for being alone; a lack of desire for close relationships; anhedonia, indifference, and emotional detachment[123]—all patently non-normative attributes. Although none of the socially anxious women whose testimonies feature in this book explicitly identified with this diagnosis, or with Laing's description of the schizoid individual, a thread which ran through all of their narratives was one of experiencing unease because of not fitting into mainstream society: adopting a false self seemed to allow them to belong. I am not the first to have spotted commonalities between social anxiety and the schizoid position. Christopher Lane, in discussing the arbitrary nature of the *DSM*'s divisions between diagnoses, asks: 'Where, for instance, did schizoid personality disorder end and social phobia begin?'[124] Phoebe's account illustrates this fuzziness, for it merges seeking to fit in with social interaction: '[W]hen I was younger I would copy my sister when she would socialise, because I didn't know how to.' In imitating her sister's normative behaviour, Phoebe was seeking not only to fit in and allay others' negative appraisals, but was arguably undertaking 'the creation of a new person'.[125]

A prime location, albeit virtual, for the creation of a new person is social media. Despite some scholars contending that the Internet allows people to express their 'true selves' more easily,[126] academics Brooke Erin Duffy and Ngai Keung Chan note that '[s]ocial media users are routinely counseled [*sic*] to cultivate their online personae with acumen and diligence' and engage in 'impression management'.[127] Ria had this to say regarding online personae:

> [T]he advent of things like Instagram [...] you're presenting a truth [...] you're presenting particular aspects [...] you're essentially making like an avatar, a projection, and it's like your idealised self.

Orbach has commented on the creation of virtual selves, noting that since the virtual world dispenses with embodiment, it dematerialises people's existence and hence facilitates the creation of 'identities, personalities and bodies that have existed until now only in one's mind's eye'.[128] Marrying this with Ria's remarks, the online persona could be construed as the digital counterpart to the false self.

Departing from social *media*, but remaining with the social, Phoebe's exposition of socialising reminds us that interactions are incredibly pertinent to theorising women's social anxiety. How do these play out once the socially anxious woman has created 'a new person'?[129] To unpack this, I call again upon Laing's false self.

Social Interaction and Laing's False Self

In order to participate in life without experiencing anxiety, Laing contends that 'being like everyone else, being someone other than oneself, playing a part, being incognito, anonymous, being nobody (psychotically, pretending to have no body) are defences that are carried through with great thoroughness in certain schizoid and schizophrenic conditions'.[130] He continues to describe a person of this type who

> [I]s, therefore, driven compulsively to seek company, but never allows himself to 'be himself' in the presence of anyone else. He avoids social anxiety by never really *being with* others. He never quite says what he means or means what he says. The part he plays is always not quite himself. He takes care to laugh when he thinks a joke is *not* funny, and look bored when he is amused. He makes friends with people he does not really like and is rather cool to those with whom he would 'really' like to be friends. No one, therefore, really knows him, or understands him. He can be *himself* in safety only in isolation, albeit with a sense of emptiness and unreality. With others, he plays an elaborate game of pretence and equivocation. His social self is felt to be false and futile.[131]

As such, and as interviewees' narratives demonstrate in due course, the false self functions as a disguise or shield for socially anxious women: if it is negatively evaluated, it does not matter, since it is not the real self.

A real, true, or inner self is a recurring concept in Laing's case studies, and it describes the self which typically remains hidden. It stands in contradistinction to a persona or false self, which is the self that interacts with the world. With that said, a number of Laing's case studies found that their real self need *not* remain hidden if they were with people they did not know.[132] Laing tells us that this is because being among strangers, where the real self is not known, renders it 'safe from penetrating remarks'.[133] By extension, if the individual were to travel to a place where they were not known, they would not experience any kind of self-consciousness or social anxiety.[134] This was apparent when I interviewed Phoebe:

> [M]eeting new people doesn't bother me [...] if I walk into a room of new people: doesn't bother me [...] I can go to like new hobbies and that doesn't bother me [...] I went to this like choir thing last night, and there was like no people I knew there: didn't bother me, at all.

In Chap. 3, recall that it was *friends*, rather than strangers, by whom Phoebe, Ellen, and Amy feared being negatively evaluated. Olivia's experience was akin to this insofar as she said: 'I'm the most socially anxious around people I know a little. They have some unknown preconceived idea of me which makes me anxious and then I'm anxious about how I'm adding to that and if it's negative.' These women all seem to experience social anxiety when they are known. In such circumstances, unfavourable evaluation would be a slight upon these women's *actual* selves, as opposed to their outward personae.

The counterpart to this phenomenon[135] is exemplified in Laing's observation that some people who are self-conscious in their everyday lives lose this trait when giving performances, such as acting: '[T]he very situation, on first reflection, one might suppose would be most difficult for them to negotiate.'[136] Phoebe's words struck a chord with this in that she reported being 'okay with public speaking'. Likewise, some of Scott's shy case studies divulged that they enjoyed acting in the theatre, since 'performing was easier when it was explicitly acknowledged that all the participants were playing parts inconsistent with their backstage selves'.[137] This certainly calls to mind my own enjoyment of theatre during my school years. Offstage, I felt that my behaviours were constrained by what others had come to expect of me, much like Farah described. Drama then offered a means by which I could transgress others' expectations without having to negotiate their reactions: however I acted on stage, I was not really being myself.

Daniella mentioned playing a part in describing how 'with everyone else I need to put up a face'. She explained: '[W]hen I'm talking to people

[...] I get a massive headache [...] another sign of social anxiety is [...] that you feel drained [...] it's an effort.' Daniella's thoughts conjure up the testimony of Rose Hughes, an autistic woman quoted in a National Autistic Society article on autism in women. Therein, Hughes describes herself as 'the master of disguise. I have always worn a mask'.[138] Likewise, other research has found 'pretending to be normal' to be a common experience of women diagnosed with autism.[139] That is not to suggest that Daniella has undiagnosed autism. Rather, it reinforces the idea that non-normativity—arising from personality type, neurodiversity, a physical health condition or experiences of mental distress—is conducive to experiencing social anxiety. Adopting a false self salves this social anxiety, for it permits our non-normative woman to conform and hence function in the world.

While Daniella spoke about needing to 'put up a face', Farah more explicitly detailed adopting a mask. She explained how this would play out at gatherings amongst peers: 'I wasn't able to talk [...] because I hate my shaking voice [...] Being [a] sort of shy person, it was a bit hard.' As such, she adopted 'a kind of strategy' where she would deliver a '[g]ood sentence, and then I couldn't say anything else, because I was shy': 'I [would] just ask a question and then get silent and make [...] chaos among people. Because you [can] always ask a kind of problematic question [laughs] and then listen to people.' In her work on shyness, Scott noted this strategy in one of her respondents who would ask 'an open-ended question that encouraged others to talk', a 'question that I know is going to take a long time to answer and is going to cause a big old debate around the table, where everyone gets involved.... So then I can sit back'.[140] In doing so, this respondent 'could move the spotlight onto [other people] and avoid the dangers of saying the wrong thing under scrutiny'.[141]

While Farah's strategy likewise serves to divert attention from her, it has other functions, as she explained: 'I could cover my shyness by [...] This mask of... Wisdom.' Contrary to her quietness causing people to 'think that I'm stupid, or I don't have anything to say' or that her reserve is 'something that's imposed on me because of... My lack of ability', Farah's strategy conveyed the image that her quietness was 'just my style'. She continued: '[I]t was like a mask [...] To pretend that it's a personality that I've chosen [...] masking, and you would be silent, and pretend that you are a good listener and just [a] kind of wise person.' Farah's description again evokes the words of Scott, who draws attention to a disconnect between what the shy 'perceive as their "real," backstage selves, who are hopelessly incompetent, and the impression of being poised and in control that they would like [to] portray'.[142]

Farah told me that she initially 'wasn't comfortable at all' in adopting her mask, but 'after a while you get used to it and I was happy about it'. This contentment with what could be described as her false self possibly results from its allowing her to participate in life in ways which she would otherwise be unable. Similarly, Laing cites one of his case studies as being uncomfortable until he could turn himself 'into some role or part which was not him, and which he felt was a suitable disguise. This enabled him to "uncouple" his "self" from his actions, and function smoothly, without anxiety'.[143] Farah's strategy may achieve something comparable, for she told me that 'each time that you are forced to be silent [...] you are not yourself [...] it's like pretending that you are someone else [...] to avoid conflict'. Like Laing's case study, who had 'always felt shy, self-conscious and vulnerable',[144] in donning her 'mask of wisdom' and remaining silent, perhaps Farah finds 'reassurance in the consideration that whatever [s]he was doing [s]he was not being [her]self'.[145]

Considering Laing's latter remark, Daniella expressed that she was herself only with her boyfriend, confessing that 'it's really hard for me to be myself with anyone else'. Daniella's deployment of her false self thus seems to be contingent on the company she keeps at any given moment. Following on from this, Laing notes that an individual may be split into 'two *or more* selves'.[146] This was evident in Scott's shy respondents, many of whom 'adapted their behavior to the demands of each situation'[147] such that 'no one ever saw their "true," backstage selves'.[148] This theme came to the fore in interviewing Farah, who explained that while her many selves had 'something—a shared thing' in common, she 'would also sometimes decide to share something with this person, and then share other things with [an]other person, rather than share everything with one person'. By dint of this variation, she reported that: 'I would always try to have my friends separately [...] you can't meet all of them together.' When I think about having different groups of my *own* friends meeting one another, I am rendered a little uneasy. If I dig deeper, this discomfort is born of my uncertainty in trying to answer the question, 'Who will I be?' I asked Farah how she would navigate such a situation herself, to which she replied, 'I don't like it and I don't do it!'

Farah's thoughts on many selves conjure up philosopher William James's statement that one has 'as many different social selves as there are distinct *groups* of persons about whose opinion he cares'.[149] Perhaps, in the words of Dr Jekyll, '[M]an will be ultimately known for a mere polity of multifarious, incongruous, and independent denizens.'[150] And, to my point about different groups of my friends meeting, James puts forth that 'there results what practically is a division of the man into several selves; and this may be a discordant splitting, as where one is afraid to let one set of his acquaintances know him as he is elsewhere'.[151]

While Farah spoke of there being something common to her many selves, if we are to draw on the poststructuralist tenet of the 'death of the subject', we might consider that 'people are socially constituted as social selves, and these social selves are historically variable rather than being a natural or fixed essence of self'.[152] That is, we might refute the notion of the self as 'a fully-constituted "subject" that stands outside context'.[153] Instead, the many selves of the socially anxious woman are produced 'through the discourses and practices of femininity [...] of our time',[154] as well as through her interactions with different (groups of) others.

The presence of many a self within us has been described as 'plurality', which is 'an umbrella term for any way in which people experience themselves as different selves, parts, or states at different times'.[155] That is, '[A]n individual can be conceptualized as a plurality of qualitatively distinct selves as well as a one.'[156] Writer and scholar Meg-John Barker's explanation of plurality is one to which many readers will be able to relate:

> People often find it easiest to recognise plurality in themselves when they reflect on how they behave in different relationships or situations. Trevor Butt's[157] research found that most people experience and express quite different character traits with different people in their lives, despite retaining a sense that they were 'being themselves' in all those relationships.[158]

Plurality will be instrumental going forward into the next section, for it is through this concept that we can understand how the selves of the socially anxious woman interact to produce an inner dialogue and, in turn, an inner critic, both of which featured prominently in participants' stories.

The Inner Worlds of Socially Anxious Women

Looking back to Chap. 2, I outlined how Jane M. Ussher and Janette Perz had identified inner critics in women experiencing PMS:[159] these were understood using self-surveillance.[160] Merging this with the gendering of emotional labour in relationships—especially the importance of 'not upsetting people'[161]—we arrive at Phoebe's testimony: 'I'd worry so much about like if I'd upset anyone [...] I get so obsessed about things I've said and things I've done, all like, "Oh God, why did I say that? [...] I bet they hate me now."'

Since such self-critique necessitates a distance from the part of the self that interacts with others, we can further comprehend this aspect of the socially anxious woman's experience if we think about her possessing a true and false self. Recall that Laing tells us that the true self is 'extremely aware of itself, and observes the false self, usually highly critically'.[162] This rang true in Farah's self-critique concerning how she appeared to others:

> I remember that there [were] lots of moments [...] when I was forced to speak and I couldn't and [...] I wasn't satisfied about my presentation, for example, even among my friends. After that I had lots of—in an obsessive way—I would think about the whole scene, a thousand times [...] remember it, and analyse it, and [...] check people's gesture[s] to guess what they think about me.

She also told me that she had

> Imaginary dialogue with people in my mind a lot [...] and sometimes in an obsessive way I would try to analyse what I've said, for example, what I could say... Or continue the conversation that I'm not satisfied about [...] when it happened in the past.

Farah's narrative draws links with Berger's exposition of a woman's being split into surveyor and surveyed. What using Laingian selves adds to this is insight into how the socially anxious woman's true self not only *surveys* but *critiques*—and its concern is not primarily the body, pace Berger, but it extends to *every aspect* of the false self.

Exploring self-critique warrants revisiting the Dissociative Disorders,[163] particularly Dissociative Identity Disorder (DID). The diagnostic criteria for DID comprise 'recurrent disruption of conscious functioning and sense of self'[164] as well as the 'fragmentation'[165] or 'division'[166] of identity which is 'characterized by two or more distinct personality states'.[167] Daniella invoked this division in discussing socialising:

> And you believe that you want to do it, it makes you happy, like, 'Ooh, that's a great idea.' Or sometimes, I would ask them, so I would be like, 'Let's go for coffee,' and then I would pull out [...] I always feel like I've

> got a split personality. Not a 'split personality' in the medical sense [...] I always have a rational side and an irrational side [...] the line is so defined, like so you can feel it.

Daniella's narrative parallels other facets of the Dissociative Disorders, particularly 'loss of personal agency'[168] and 'feeling like one's body or actions are not one's own'.[169] Indeed, this altered sense of self[170] can be 'accompanied by a feeling that these attitudes, emotions, and behaviours — even one's body — are "not mine" and/or are "not under my control"'.[171] This echoes Ussher and Perz's exposition of women's experiencing premenstrual negative affect as 'not me'.[172] Daniella's account of struggling with binge eating further resonated with this disconnect: '[W]hen I want to binge. My irrational side—I can feel the difference. So my rational side is trying to fight against it and the irrational side, it just goes, "Nah, mate." [...] [Y]ou can feel the two clashing.'

This segment of Daniella's story relates to other feminist work on PMS besides that of Ussher and Perz. Recall from Chap. 2 that Chrisler found the narrative '"Jekyll & Hyde", "me/not me," "PMS-self/real-self"' to be present in PMS self-help books.[173] In addition, several studies have found the tendency among heterosexual women to position 'PMS as something separate from themselves, as "not me", or as the "PMS self"'.[174] Amy conceptualised her mental distress in this manner, calling compartmentalisation 'an important element of coping [...] a coping mechanism'. For Amy, this facilitated 'understanding which responses and behaviours and thoughts are coming from the anxiety place, are coming from the depression place'. In turn, she found herself referring to 'depression brain' and 'anxiety brain' in contradistinction to her 'logic brain', telling me, '[T]hat's another way of thinking about it [...] internally it's as separate brains'. As such, she described her mental distress as 'a separate part of me':

> It gives me an opportunity to say, 'Right, that's the illness talking, so let's put it over here and acknowledge it but also recognise that [...] it's not coming from my logic brain' [...] And then I can use my logic brain to work through it.

What also emerged from Amy's account was that she experienced mental distress as voices. This again speaks to the diagnostic criteria for DID,[175] which describe how one experiences 'recurrent, inexplicable intrusions into their conscious functioning and sense of self',[176] such as 'perceptions of voices'.[177] These voices may be 'experienced as multiple, perplexing, independent thought streams over which the individual experiences no control';[178] they may be 'persecutory and derogatory'[179] and 'personified, internally communicative inner voices'.[180] Amy gave the following examples: 'My depression said I couldn't get out of bed today [...] Depression says: don't do anything. And anxiety says: you need to do everything!'

In a manner akin to Daniella's account of binge eating, Amy's narrative also drew links with the lack of control over one's attitudes, emotions, and behaviours which is described by DID's diagnostic criteria.[181] That is, she explained that her mental distress has its own agency, since her social anxiety 'shows up wherever it wants to'. Likewise, her depression/anxiety is

> [L]ike a monster, just like hanging out with you, like a demon on your shoulder, kind of thing, where sometimes it just decides, 'This is what today is going to be,' and sometimes you just have to listen to it.

This excerpt of Amy's account has much in common with women's positioning of pre-menstrual 'symptoms' as outside of themselves—a positioning which helped these women to avoid 'an assault on the self'.[182] Perhaps this is also the case for Daniella, who, in light of norms surrounding sociability, agrees to attend social events. Attributing her reneging to her 'irrational side' allows her to avoid an assault on *her* self. For Amy, '[c]ompartmentalising into "anxiety brain" or "depression brain"' is analogous. Much like her subscription to the chemical imbalance model, she explained that compartmentalising 'allows me a distance to not shame myself', since it makes her mental distress 'separate from my conscious brain. And that is a tool for removing the burden of responsibility from my own logical thoughts'. As opposed to Amy's separation from certain parts of herself being pathological—as the *DSM-5*'s conception of DID would suggest—it helps her to cope when her feelings are out of kilter with those which society deems normative.

Having reviewed participants' narratives on inner critics, splits in their selves, and feelings of detachment from their bodies, there is patent overlap with the diagnostic criteria for the Dissociative Disorders. I have proposed that, given cultural attitudes towards women—especially their bodies—and women's socialisation, any resulting dissociation and depersonalisation are quite understandable. This supposition becomes more viable when we chart exactly how most women learn to view their bodies and their selves: from the position of outsiders. Coupling this with Amy's experience of dissociation as a positive phenomenon therefore begs the question as to whether these experiences constitute 'disorders'. On this point, Barker notes that DID—previously called 'Multiple Personality Disorder' in psychiatry—is often experienced negatively, since

> [I]t's stigmatised to the extent that it's listed in the books of 'psychiatric disorders' [...] and represented in hugely stigmatising ways in popular culture: movies and TV shows almost exclusively depict it as a form of madness and as dangerous. Pretty much any plural person shown in the mainstream media has a self who is a serial killer. Think about movies like *Identity* and *Split*.[183]

Recall that Daniella sought to distance herself from representations such as these in telling me, 'I always feel like I've got a split personality', being sure to add the caveat, '[n]ot a "split personality" in the medical sense'. Barker thus advocates for a more positive framing of this experience and renames it 'plural selves' or, as I touched on earlier, 'plurality', noting that those who identify thus 'generally find [it] a pretty positive experience'.[184] Barker even identifies one of their own selves as their 'inner critic', whom they call 'Beastie'.

In addition to Barker's work, there is existing scholarship on plurality and much has elements in common with Laing's writings. For one, psychotherapist John Rowan, in his co-edited volume *The Plural Self*, gives an account of the plural self's development which is reminiscent of Laing's, and Winnicott's, exposition of the genesis of the infant's true-false self dyad.[185] Crucially, in Rowan's work, the deployment of the false self is framed as 'a means of surviving potentially annihilating experiences'.[186] In the same volume, psychologist Leon Rappoport and colleagues contend that postmodern society demands a plural self owing to 'rapid social change [which] necessitates a readiness to access alternative views of the self [...] transformation, flux and plurality have become the celebrated values of our time'.[187] The plural self is thus presented as a rational, even necessary, response to life in postmodern society, and therein we find the implicit question as to whether these experiences really constitute illness.

Most relevant for this chapter's theoretical reliance on Laing's selves, and his conception of schizophrenia as a 'metanoiac voyage',[188] Barker contends that 'exploring [...] plurality, rather than ignoring or resisting it, could be a valuable therapeutic, spiritual, and/or political endeavour'.[189] Relatedly, author Ruth-Inge Heinze questions Western culture's insistence that plurality is abnormal or pathological. She draws on almost four decades of cross-cultural fieldwork, largely in Southeast Asia, which features 'case-examples of spirit mediumship, glossolalia, automatic writing, possession trances, and dramatic performance'.[190] In so doing, she challenges the 'modernist, occidental assumption of a unified self'[191] and argues that experiencing many selves 'may be considered quite acceptable – and frequently valuable – in other cultural contexts'.[192] Perhaps then, like SAD in women, there is room to consider plurality—or its pathologised form, DID—in women through the lens of the culture-bound syndrome (CBS).

With the exception of Laing's work, a theoretical void in extant scholarship on plurality is its omission of social anxiety. The *DSM-5*'s diagnostic criteria for DID, and indeed Depersonalization/Derealization Disorder, bear no mention of SAD, whereas this chapter has demonstrated their connectedness. That is not to say that all of the women I interviewed have a Dissociative Disorder. Rather, the overlap between SAD and a purportedly *un*related diagnostic category again points to the arbitrary nature of these diagnostic categories themselves. It also bespeaks the central flaw in the *DSM-5*'s contention that these diagnostic categories represent *diagnoses*, as opposed to *descriptions*. Moreover, in bringing participants' narratives to the fore, this book suggests that the inner worlds of socially anxious women; how they experience social anxiety; how they make sense of it; and how they conceptualise it, are not well understood. Indeed, psy science discourses have thus far made little attempt to render these very gendered experiences explicable, nor take heed of women's own accounts. This book has begun to remedy this absence.

Notes

1. My emphasis.
2. Michel Foucault, *Discipline and Punish* [*Surveiller et Punir*] trans. Alan Sheridan (Harmondsworth: Penguin, 1991[1975]).
3. Michel Foucault, *Power/Knowledge: Selected Interviews and other Writings, 1972–1977*, ed. by Colin Gordon (New York: Pantheon Books, 1980), p. 131.
4. John Berger, *Ways of Seeing* (Harmondsworth: Penguin, 2008), p. 41.
5. Ibid., p. 40.
6. Ibid., pp. 40–41.
7. Susie Orbach, *Fat Is a Feminist Issue* (London: Arrow Books Limited, 1986), p. 30.

8. Susie Orbach, *Bodies* (New York: Picador, 2009), p. 108.
9. Meenakshi Gigi Durham, 'Articulating Adolescent Girls' Resistance to Patriarchal Discourse in Popular Media', *Women's Studies in Communication*, 22.2 (1999), 210–29 https://doi.org/10.1080/07491409.1999.10162421 p. 222, cited in Valerie Steeves, '"Pretty and Just a Little Bit Sexy, I Guess": Publicity, Privacy, and the Pressure To Perform "Appropriate" Femininity on Social Media', in *EGirls, ECitizens: Putting Technology, Theory and Policy into Dialogue with Girls' and Young Women's Voices*, ed. by Valerie Steeves and Jane Bailey (Ottawa, Ontario: University of Ottawa Press, 2015), 153–73, p. 169.
10. Berger, *Ways of Seeing*, p. 40.
11. Susan Sontag, *New York Review of Books*, 18 April 1974.
12. Angela McRobbie, 'Notes on the Perfect: Competitive Femininity in Neoliberal Times', *Australian Feminist Studies*, 30.83 (2015), 3–20 https://doi.org/10.1080/08164649.2015.1011485 p. 7.
13. Ronald David Laing, *The Divided Self: An Existential Study in Sanity and Madness* (London: Tavistock Publications Ltd., 1965), p. 174.
14. Laura Mulvey, 'Visual Pleasure and Narrative Cinema', *Screen*, 16.3 (1975), 6–18 https://doi.org/10.1007/978-1-349-19798-9_3
15. Janet Holland, Caroline Ramazanoglu, Sue Sharpe, and Rachel Thomson, *The Male in the Head: Young People, Heterosexuality and Power* (London: The Tufnell Press, 1998), p. 11.
16. Ibid., p. 188.
17. Kathy Deliovsky, 'Normative White Femininity: Race, Gender and the Politics of Beauty', *Atlantis: Critical Studies in Gender, Culture and Social Justice*, 33.1 (2008), 49–59 https://journals.msvu.ca/index.php/atlantis/article/view/429 [accessed 30 January 2023] p. 57. My emphases.
18. Holland et al. *The Male in the Head*, p. 173.
19. Sandra Lee Bartky, 'Foucault, Femininity, and the Modernization of Patriarchal Power', in *The Politics of Women's Bodies: Sexuality, Appearance, and Behavior*, ed. by Rose Weitz (New York and Oxford: Oxford University Press, 1998), 25–45, p. 34.
20. Orbach, *Bodies*, p. 108.
21. Margaret Attwood, *The Robber Bride* (New York, Doubleday, 1993), p. 388.
22. Susie Orbach, *Hunger Strike: Starving amidst Plenty* (London and New York: Karnac, 2005), p. 28.
23. Ibid., p. 16.
24. Ibid.
25. Joan C. Chrisler and Ingrid Johnston-Robledo, 'Woman's Embodied Self: An Introduction', in *Woman's Embodied Self: Feminist Perspectives on*

Identity and Image, ed. by J. C. Chrisler and I. Johnston-Robledo (Washington, DC: American Psychological Association, 2018), 3–14, p. 12.
26. Orbach, *Hunger Strike*, p. 16.
27. Ibid., p. 28.
28. Susan Bordo, *Unbearable Weight: Feminism, Western Culture, and the Body*, 10th edn (Berkeley: University of California Press, 2003). Deliovsky, 'Normative White Femininity', p. 57.
29. Orbach, *Hunger Strike*, p. 16.
30. Ibid., p. 28.
31. Holland et al., *The Male in the Head*, p. 109.
32. American Psychiatric Association, *Diagnostic and Statistical Manual of Mental Disorders* [*DSM-5*] (Washington, DC: American Psychiatric Association Publishing, 2013) https://ebookcentral.proquest.com/lib/bham/reader.action?docID=1811753 [accessed 6 January 2021] p. 291.
33. Ibid., p. 273.
34. Emily Martin, *The Woman in the Body* (Milton Keynes: Open University Press, 1989), p. 89, cited in Holland et al., *The Male in the Head*, p. 109.
35. Incidentally, 'Depersonalization/Derealization Disorder' is *not* reported as being 'co-morbid' with SAD by the *DSM-5*. At the time of writing, extant literature provides no reference to any link between the 'Dissociative Disorders' and 'SAD' aside from one qualitative study and one psychological study. These are, respectively:
Matthias Michal, Johannes Kaufhold, Ralph Grabhorn, Karsten Krakow, Gerd Overbeck, and Thomas Heidenreich, 'Depersonalization and Social Anxiety', *The Journal of Nervous and Mental Disease*, 193.9 (2005), 629–32 https://doi.org/10.1097/01.nmd.0000178038.87332.ec and Juergen Hoyer, David Braeuer, Stephen Crawcour, Elisabeth Klumbies, and Clemens Kirschbaum, 'Depersonalization/Derealization during Acute Social Stress in Social Phobia', *Journal of Anxiety Disorders*, 27.2 (2013), 178–87 https://doi.org/10.1016/j.janxdis.2013.01.002
36. Chloë Taylor, 'Female Sexual Dysfunction, Feminist Sexology, and the Psychiatry of the Normal', *Feminist Studies*, 41.2 (2015), 259–92 https://doi.org/10.15767/feministstudies.41.2.259 p. 286.
37. Laing, *The Divided Self*, p. 19.
38. Orbach, *Bodies*, p. 151.
39. Ibid., p. 111.
40. Deliovsky, 'Normative White Femininity', p. 56.
41. Orbach, *Bodies*, p. 168.
42. Chrisler and Johnston-Robledo, 'Woman's Embodied Self', p. 4.
43. Orbach, *Hunger Strike*, p. 4.

44. Ambrose Bierce, *The Devil's Dictionary* (New York: Albert and Charles Boni, 1935[1911]).
    Miriam Greenspan, *A New Approach to Women and Therapy* (New York, NY: McGraw-Hill, 1983).
    All cited in Chrisler and Johnston-Robledo, 'Woman's Embodied Self', p. 3.
45. Susan Sontag, 'The Double Standard of Aging', *in Psychology of Women*, ed. by J. Williams (New York: Academic Press, 1979), 462–78, cited in Chrisler and Johnston-Robledo, 'Woman's Embodied Self', p. 4.
46. Orbach, *Hunger Strike*, p. 4.
47. Ibid., p. 107.
48. Morag MacSween, *Anorexic Bodies: A Feminist and Sociological Perspective on Anorexia Nervosa* (London and New York, Routledge, 1993), p. 193.
49. Laura T. Hamilton, Elizabeth A. Armstrong, J. Lotus Seeley, and Elizabeth M. Armstrong, 'Hegemonic Femininities and Intersectional Domination', *Sociological Theory*, 37. 4 (2019), 315–41 https://doi.org/10.1177/0735275119888248 p. 315.
50. Orbach, *Hunger Strike*, p. 95.
51. Ashley M. Shaw, Kiara R. Timpano, Tanya B. Tran, and Jutta Joormann, 'Correlates of Facebook Usage Patterns: The Relationship between Passive Facebook Use, Social Anxiety Symptoms, and Brooding', *Computers in Human Behavior*, 48 (2015), 575–80 https://doi.org/10.1016/j.chb.2015.02.003
52. Sang Yup Lee, 'How Do People Compare Themselves with Others on Social Network Sites?: The Case of Facebook', *Computers in Human Behavior*, 32 (2014), 253–60 https://doi.org/10.1016/j.chb.2013.12.009 p. 253.
53. Katerina Lup, Leora Trub, and Lisa Rosenthal, 'Instagram #Instasad?: Exploring Associations among Instagram Use, Depressive Symptoms, Negative Social Comparison, and Strangers Followed', *Cyberpsychology, Behavior, and Social Networking*, 18.5 (2015), 247–52 https://doi.org/10.1089/cyber.2014.0560
    Mai-Ly N. Steers, Robert E. Wickham, and Linda K. Acitelli, 'Seeing Everyone Else's Highlight Reels: How Facebook Usage Is Linked to Depressive Symptoms', *Journal of Social and Clinical Psychology*, 33.8 (2014), 701–31 https://doi.org/10.1521/jscp.2014.33.8.701
    Lee, 'How Do People Compare Themselves with Others…?'.
    Brian A. Feinstein, Rachel Hershenberg, Vickie Bhatia, Jessica A. Latack, Nathalie Meuwly, and Joanne Davila, 'Negative Social Comparison on Facebook and Depressive Symptoms: Rumination as a Mechanism', *Psychology of Popular Media Culture*, 2.3 (2013), 161–70 https://doi.org/10.1037/a0033111

All cited in Elizabeth M. Seabrook, Margaret L. Kern, and Nikki S. Rickard, 'Social Networking Sites, Depression, and Anxiety: A Systematic Review', *JMIR Mental Health*, 3.4 (2016), e50 https://doi.org/10.2196/mental.5842 p. 8.

54. Hamilton et al., 'Hegemonic Femininities', p. 322.
55. Orbach, *Bodies*, p. 166.
56. Catherine Baker-Pitts, 'Symptoms or Solution? The Relational Meaning of Cosmetic Surgery for Women' (unpublished dissertation, New York University, 2008), cited in Orbach, *Bodies*, pp. 102–03.
57. Wendy Chapkis, *Beauty Secrets: Women and the Politics of Appearance* (Boston: South End Press, 1986), cited in Deliovsky, 'Normative White Femininity', p. 57.
58. Baker-Pitts, 'Symptoms or Solution?', cited in Orbach, *Bodies*, pp. 102–03.
59. Peter D. Kramer, *Listening to Prozac* (London: Fourth Estate, 1994), p. xvi.
60. Ibid., p. 143.
61. Berger, *Ways of Seeing*, p. 40.
62. Laing, *The Divided Self.*
63. Joan C. Chrisler, 'How To Regain Your Control and Balance: The "Pop" Approach to PMS', Manuscript under review (2001), cited in Joan C. Chrisler and Paula Caplan, 'The Strange Case of Dr. Jekyll and Ms. Hyde: How PMS Became a Cultural Phenomenon and a Psychiatric Disorder', *Annual Review of Sex Research*, 13:1 (2002), 274–306 https://doi.org/10.1080/10532528.2002.10559807 p. 276, 288.
64. Robert Louis Stevenson, *The Strange Case of Dr Jekyll and Mr Hyde* (Hertfordshire: Wordsworth Editions, Ltd., 1993), pp. 48–49.
65. Although extensive discussion of psychosis is beyond the scope of this work, in brief, it can be described as: '[W]hen people lose some contact with reality. This might involve seeing or hearing things that other people cannot see or hear (hallucinations) and believing things that are not actually true (delusions).' See NHS, *Overview - Psychosis* (2019) https://www.nhs.uk/mental-health/conditions/psychosis/overview/ [accessed 5 June 2023].
66. Orbach, *Bodies*, pp. 81–82.
67. Ibid., p. 81.
68. Ibid.
69. Ibid., p. 82.
70. Ibid.
71. Orbach, *Hunger Strike*, p. 70.
72. Orbach, *Bodies*, p. 82.
73. Ibid.
74. Ibid.

75. Orbach, *Hunger Strike*, p. 70.
76. Orbach, *Bodies*, p. 82.
77. Laing, *The Divided Self*, p. 190.
78. Ibid., p. 69.
79. Ibid.
80. Ibid.
81. APA, *DSM-5*, p. 293.
82. Ibid., p. 303.
83. Ibid., p. 302.
84. Laing, *The Divided Self*, p. 117.
85. Ibid.
86. Ibid., p. 112.
87. Ibid., p. 74.
88. Orbach, *Hunger Strike*, p. 87.
89. Richard A. Wasserstrom, 'Racism, Sexism and Preferential Treatment: An Approach to the Topics', *UCLA Law Review*, 24 (1977), 581–622 https://leonletwin.files.wordpress.com/2016/06/1977-02-00-wasserstrom-racism-sexism-and-preferential-treatment-ucla-l-rev-ocr.pdf [accessed 22 June 2023] p. 588, cited in Kimberlé Crenshaw, 'Demarginalizing the Intersection of Race and Sex: A Black Feminist Critique of Antidiscrimination Doctrine, Feminist Theory and Antiracist Politics', *University of Chicago Legal Forum*, 1.8 (1989), 139–67 http://chicagounbound.uchicago.edu/uclf/vol1989/iss1/8 p. 155.
90. Ibid.
91. Ibid.
92. Chrisler and Johnston-Robledo, 'Woman's Embodied Self', p. 11.
93. Virginia Woolf, 'The Professions of Women', in *Virginia Woolf: Selected Essays*, ed. by David Bradshaw (New York: Oxford University Press, 2008), 140–45, p. 141.
94. Lisa Downing, *Selfish Women* (Abingdon, Oxon; New York, NY: Routledge, 2019), p. 1.
95. Holland et al., *The Male in the Head*, p. 112.
96. Ibid.
97. Orbach, *Hunger Strike*, pp. 143–44.
98. Downing, *Selfish Women*, p. 1.
99. Susie Orbach and Luise Eichenbaum, *Understanding Women* (Harmondsworth: Penguin, 1985), p. 7.
100. Orbach, *Hunger Strike*, pp. 143–44.
101. Laing, *The Divided Self*, p. 98.
102. Orbach, *Fat Is a Feminist Issue*, p. 88.
103. Downing, *Selfish Women*, p. 1.
104. Orbach, *Hunger Strike*, p. 24.

105. Ibid.
106. Ibid., p. 63.
107. Steeves, '"Pretty and Just a Little Bit Sexy"', p. 165. My emphasis.
108. Ibid.
109. Marion Milner, *A Life of One's Own* (Taylor and Francis Group, 2011) https://ebookcentral.proquest.com/lib/bham/reader.action?docID=672403 [accessed 24 September 2020] p. 89.
110. Elaine Showalter, *The Female Malady: Women, Madness, and English Culture* (New York: Pantheon, 1985), p. 231.
111. Orbach, *Hunger Strike*, p. 9.
112. Dana Crowley Jack and Diana Dill, 'The Silencing the Self Scale: Schemas of Intimacy with Depression in Women', *Psychology of Women Quarterly*, 16.1 (1992), 97–106 https://doi.org/10.1111/j.1471-6402.1992.tb00242.x p. 98.
    Jane M. Ussher and Janette Perz, 'PMS as a Gendered Illness Linked to the Construction and Relational Experience of Hetero-femininity', *Sex Roles*, 68 (2013), 132–50 https://doi.org/10.1007/s11199-011-9977-5 p. 135.
113. Jack and Dill, 'The Silencing the Self Scale', cited in Ussher and Perz, 'PMS as a Gendered Illness', p. 135.
114. Laing, *The Divided Self*, p. 99.
115. Ferenczi, 'The Nosology of Male Homosexuality', *Contributions to Psychoanalysis*, (1916), cited in Joan Riviere, 'Womanliness as a Masquerade', *International Journal of Psychoanalysis*, 10 (1929), 303–13, p. 303.
116. Riviere, 'Womanliness as a Masquerade', pp. 303, 306.
117. McRobbie, 'Notes on the Perfect', p. 17.
118. Arlie Russell Hochschild, *The Managed Heart: Commercialization of Human Feeling*, 3rd edn (University of California Press, 2012) https://ebookcentral.proquest.com/lib/bham/reader.action?docID=870020&query=Hochschild%2C+the+Managed+Heart [accessed 31 July 2020].
119. Downing, *Selfish Women*, p. 102.
120. Laing, *The Divided Self*, p. 166.
121. Susie Scott, 'The Shell, the Stranger and the Competent Other: Towards a Sociology of Shyness', *Sociology*, 38.1 (2004), 121–37 https://doi.org/10.1177/0038038504039364 p. 125.
122. Laing, *The Divided Self*, p. 192, cited in Scott, 'The Shell, the Stranger and the Competent Other', p. 125.
123. APA, *DSM-5*, p. 653.
124. Christopher Lane, *Shyness: How Normal Behavior Became a Sickness* (Yale University Press, 2007) https://ebookcentral.proquest.com/lib/bham/reader.action?docID=3420940 [accessed 6 January 2021] p. 92.
125. Orbach, *Hunger Strike*, p. 131.

126. John A. Bargh, Katelyn Y. A. McKenna, and Grainne M. Fitzsimons, 'Can You See the Real Me? Activation and Expression of the "True Self" on the Internet', *Journal of Social Issues*, 58.1 (2002), 33–48 https://doi.org/10.1111/1540-4560.00247
127. Brooke Erin Duffy and Ngai Keung Chan, '"You Never really Know Who's Looking": Imagined Surveillance across Social Media Platforms', *New Media and Society*, 21.1 (2019), 119–38 https://doi.org/10.1177/1461444818791318
128. Orbach, *Bodies*, p. 97.
129. Orbach, *Hunger Strike*, p. 131.
130. Laing, *The Divided Self*, p. 11.
131. Ibid., p. 114.
132. Ibid., p. 73.
133. Ibid., p. 139.
134. Ibid., pp. 128, 139.
135. I have previously linked this to women's social anxiety. See Katie Masters, 'An Analysis of Women and Social Anxiety Disorder from the Perspectives of Feminism and Anti-psychiatry' (unpublished Master of Research thesis, University of Birmingham, 2016).
136. Laing, *The Divided Self*, p. 107.
137. Susie Scott, 'The Red, Shaking Fool: Dramaturgical Dilemmas in Shyness', *Symbolic Interaction*, 28.1 (2005), 91–110 https://doi.org/10.1525/si.2005.28.1.91 p. 100.
138. National Autistic Society, *How Do Women and Girls Experience Autism?* (2018) https://www.autism.org.uk/about/what-is/gender/stories.aspx [accessed 31 July 2020].
139. Sarah Bargiela, Robyn Steward, and William Mandy, 'The Experiences of Late-diagnosed Women with Autism Spectrum Conditions: An Investigation of the Female Autism Phenotype', *Journal of Autism and Developmental Disorders*, 46.10 (2016), 3281–94 https://doi.org/10.1007/s10803-016-2872-8
140. Scott, 'The Red, Shaking Fool', p. 104.
141. Ibid.
142. Ibid., p. 101.
143. Laing, *The Divided Self*, p. 127.
144. Ibid., p. 71.
145. Ibid.
146. Ibid., p. 17. My emphasis.
147. Scott, 'The Red, Shaking Fool', p. 98.
148. Ibid.
149. William James, *Psychology* (New York: Henry Holt and Company, 1893), p. 179.

150. Stevenson, *The Strange Case of Dr Jekyll and Mr Hyde*, p. 49.
151. James, *Psychology*, p. 180.
152. Holland et al., *The Male in the Head*, p. 28.
153. Morthaur, *One Year on the Web: Some Thoughts on Fractalus* (2015) http://fractalus.org/essays/one_year_p0.php cited in Kristin Bumiller, 'Quirky Citizens: Autism, Gender, and Reimagining Disability', *Signs: Journal of Women in Culture and Society*, 33.4 (2008), 967–91 https://doi.org/10.1086/528848 p. 984.
154. Holland et al., *The Male in the Head*, p. 28.
155. Meg-John Barker, 'Plural Selves, Queer, and Comics', *Journal of Graphic Novels and Comics*, 11.4 (2020), 463–74 https://doi.org/10.1080/21504857.2020.1774403 p. 464.
156. John Rowan and Mick Cooper, 'Introduction: Self-plurality: The One and the Many', in *The Plural Self: Multiplicity in Everyday Life*, ed. by John Rowan and Mick Cooper (London; Thousand Oaks; New Delhi: Sage, 1999) 1–10, pp. 1–2.
157. Trevor Butt, *Understanding People* (London: Macmillan International Higher Education, 2003).
158. Barker, 'Plural Selves, Queer, and Comics', p. 464.
159. Ussher and Perz, 'PMS as a Gendered Illness', p. 136.
160. Ibid., p. 138.
161. Jean Grimshaw, *Philosophy and Feminist Thinking* (Minneapolis: University of Minnesota Press, 1986), p. 196.
162. Laing, *The Divided Self*, p. 74.
163. APA, *DSM-5*, pp. 291–308.
164. Ibid.
165. Ibid., p. 291.
166. Ibid., p. 296.
167. Ibid., p. 292.
168. Ibid., p. 293.
169. Ibid., p. 292.
170. Ibid.
171. Ibid., p. 293.
172. Jane M. Ussher, 'The Role of Premenstrual Dysphoric Disorder in the Subjectification of Women', *Journal of Medical Humanities*, 24 (2003), 131–46 https://doi.org/10.1023/A:1021366001305 cited in Ussher and Perz, 'PMS as a Gendered Illness', p. 140.
173. Chrisler, 'How To Regain Your Control and Balance', cited in Chrisler and Caplan, 'The Strange Case of Dr. Jekyll and Ms. Hyde', pp. 276, 288.
174. Lisa Cosgrove, 'Crying out Loud: Understanding Women's Emotional Distress as both Lived Experience and Social Construction', *Feminism and Psychology*, 10.2 (2000), 247–67 https://doi.org/10.1177/0959353500010002004

Janet Lee and Jennifer Sasser-Coen, *Blood Stories: Menarche and the Politics of the Female Body in Contemporary US Society* (New York: Routledge, 1996).
Jane M. Ussher, 'Premenstrual Syndrome and Self-policing: Ruptures in Self-silencing Leading to Increased Self-surveillance and Blaming of the Body', *Social Theory and Health*, 2 (2004), 254–72 https://doi.org/10.1057/palgrave.sth.8700032
Jane M. Ussher, Myra S. Hunter, and S. J. Browne, 'Good, Bad or Dangerous To Know: Representations of Femininity in Narrative Accounts of PMS', in *Culture and Psychology*, ed. by Corinne Squire (Falmer: Routledge, 2000), 87–99.
All cited in Ussher and Perz, 'PMS as a Gendered Illness', p. 136.

175. APA, *DSM-5*.
176. Ibid., p. 292.
177. Ibid., p. 293.
178. Ibid.
179. Ibid., p. 297.
180. Ibid., p. 296.
181. Ibid., p. 293.
182. Ussher, 'The Role of Premenstrual Dysphoric Disorder', cited in Ussher and Perz, 'PMS as a Gendered Illness', p. 140.
183. Meg-John Barker, *Plural Selves FAQ* (2019) https://www.rewriting-the-rules.com/self/plural-selves-faq/ [accessed 31 July 2020].
184. Ibid.
185. John Rowan, 'The Normal Development of Subpersonalities', in Rowan and Cooper, *The Plural Self*, 11–27.
186. Rowan, 'The Normal Development of Subpersonalities', cited in John Rowan and Mick Cooper, 'Introduction: Self-plurality: The One and the Many', in Rowan and Cooper, *The Plural Self*, 1–10, p. 4.
187. Leon Rappoport, Steve Baumgardner, and George Boone, 'Postmodern Culture and the Plural Self', in *The Plural Self*, 93–106, cited in Rowan and Cooper, 'Introduction', p. 5.
188. Ronald David Laing, 'Metanoia: Some Experiences at Kingsley Hall, London', in *Going Crazy: The Radical Therapy of R. D. Laing and Others*, ed. by Hendrik M. Ruitenbeek (New York, Bantam Books, 1972), p. 12.
189. Barker, 'Plural Selves', p. 463.
190. Ruth-Inge Heinze, 'Multiplicity in Cross-cultural Perspective', in *The Plural Self*, 151–67, cited in Rowan and Cooper, 'Introduction', p. 6.
191. Rowan and Cooper, 'Introduction', p. 6.
192. Ibid.

CHAPTER 7

Conclusion

In interviewing fellow socially anxious women, I have been struck by, and even sometimes surprised at, the extent to which their experiences paralleled my own. Perhaps, until writing this book, I had little understanding of how other women experienced social anxiety—I had thought that a lot of my experiences were particular to me. I thus wonder whether this perception extends to other socially anxious women, and whether the feelings of isolation that it fosters fuel social anxiety further. On the flip side, there may be comfort to be drawn from understanding other women's experiences—experiences which, we may find, are not so different from our own.

My own positionality has no doubt brought the linkage between participants' stories and my own perspective to the fore, as well as shaping the book as a whole. For instance, my own viewpoint has influenced the questions I asked during interviews, the points on which I chose to follow up, and how I interpreted participants' testimonies. With that said, while interviewees' accounts mirrored my own views in some ways, their standpoints diverged from mine in others—their subscription to the chemical imbalance model comes to mind. Yet, regardless of whether their viewpoints concurred with my own, I have endeavoured to remain true to their perspectives and place their narratives at the very heart of this book. I also note that, irrespective of my involvement in forming the book's overarching argument, the continuity which ran through *all* of the women's stories

K. Masters, *Feminist and Anti-Psychiatry Perspectives on 'Social Anxiety Disorder'*,
https://doi.org/10.1007/978-3-031-48707-1_7

cannot be ignored: at times, they all seemed to relate similar experiences but in different ways.

Overview of the Book

The research on which the book is premised finds a place alongside other work which problematises gendered psychiatric diagnoses using critical methods.[1] Specifically, this book contributes to extant scholarship by conceptualising Social Anxiety Disorder (SAD) in women as a culture-bound syndrome (CBS) whose (pharmacological) treatment rests on cultural values: namely, normative white femininity in twenty-first-century Britain. Moreover, participants' narratives communicated that their social anxiety was an understandable response to the circumstances in which they often found themselves—a response which has been subject to medicalisation. Yet, while an SAD diagnosis was sometimes felt to pathologise, in other cases it formed a 'reverse discourse':[2] that is, this pathologisation was turned on its head and the diagnostic label functioned as a useful tool which facilitated these women's self-understanding.

This book has seen the development of three pivotal arguments, which I will now reiterate. Firstly, non-normativity is central to the socially anxious woman's experience and may assume many forms. It ranges from what psychiatry calls 'co-morbidities'—'mental disorders' and 'Neurodevelopmental Disorders'—through to physical health conditions, temperament, and body type. Exploring how society treats non-normative women reveals just why these non-normativities are so conducive to women's experiencing social anxiety.

The second argument is that SAD is not a disease entity in the way that the *DSM-5* presents. For women, the socially anxious experience invokes elements from many of the *DSM-5*'s other diagnostic categories—Eating Disorders, Selective Mutism, Generalised Anxiety Disorder, Avoidant Personality Disorder, and the Dissociative Disorders, to name but a few. This speaks to the lack of clear-cut demarcation between diagnostic categories which, in turn, supports the contention that these diagnoses are not discrete illnesses caused by underlying (biological) pathology, as psychiatry holds. By contrast, their messy entanglement, exemplified by participants' testimonies, problematises the discrete diagnostic category 'Social Anxiety Disorder' in women. By extension, it problematises the *DSM-5*, and psychiatry, as arbiters of (women's) madness.

Thirdly, this book lays bare how gender inequalities and ideologies contribute to social factors which have a more significant role to play in women's experiences of social anxiety than psychiatric discourses tell us. That is, women's socialisation fosters feelings of inadequacy in tandem with creating separateness from the self. This promotes the cultivation of a pleasing, outward self which conforms to gendered expectations—at the expense of the true self and its wants and needs—in order to stave off negative evaluation. In sum, bringing to light the impact of exogenous contributors aids in refuting the individual pathology model as applied to women (self-)diagnosed with SAD.

Impact and Significance

In providing a platform for the voices of women (self-)diagnosed with SAD, the power to define this 'disorder' is shifted from the medical professional to these women themselves. The discord which has then been ascertained by placing their narratives into dialogue with diagnostic criteria calls the diagnosis and treatment of socially anxious women into question. That is, by devoting attention to the importance of social factors in the development of women's SAD, this book departs from prior work on women's overrepresentation among those experiencing this form of mental distress. As such, it provides a corrective to biologically reductionist, medicalised, and gender biased accounts—often premised on individual pathology—which have sought to explain this gender imbalance.

Therefore, this book, dealing with the already 'neglected anxiety disorder',[3] constitutes an important addition to existing scholarship. It sits alongside a body of research which views gendered psychiatric diagnoses through a feminist lens. Further to this, it makes a significant contribution to the sociology of (mental) health and illness insofar as its focus is on the social, external, and structural factors contributing to SAD—and, to a lesser extent, associated forms of mental distress—in women.

Where Do We Go from Here?

While this book has problematised the medicalisation of women's social anxiety, a fraught issue remains: does the SAD label hold any utility and is there anything worth salvaging? These questions cannot easily, or succinctly, be answered with broad brush strokes. A starting point, however, might be found in the words of Paula J. Caplan. In her exploration of veterans' feelings and experiences in relation to the PTSD diagnosis, she poses the following questions: 'Does this seem to be a mental illness? If so, why? And what is gained and lost by calling or not calling it a mental illness?'[4]

From speaking with other socially anxious women, I have formed the view that SAD should only be construed as a 'mental illness' insofar as the women it 'affects' conceptualise it as such. At one end of the spectrum, we had Farah and Ellen, both of whom challenged the notion that their social anxiety was a 'disorder'. Elsewhere, I elaborate on Farah's viewpoint in this regard, wherein she describes using her experiences of social anxiety for self-reflection; to learn about herself; and as an impetus to create art.[5] At the other end of the spectrum, we had Amy and Phoebe. Evoking Foucault's 'reverse discourse', both of these women expressed that psychiatric diagnosis offered a means by which they could make sense of their experiences.

Where the SAD label *is* found to have utility, we should heed Sami Timimi's concerns about 'importing the diagnostic model from general medicine'.[6] Timimi makes the case that '[f]or a diagnostic system to establish itself as scientifically useful, its categories should be able to "carve nature at its joints"'.[7] Throughout this work, I have argued that the *DSM-5*'s 'Social Anxiety Disorder', and indeed its other diagnostic categories, *do not* satisfy Timimi's criterion. As such, shoehorning experiences of mental distress into 'simplistic, diagnosis-driven protocols' constitutes, in the words of Timimi, 'dumbing-down' of what psychiatry should seek to provide. And psychiatry should seek to provide 'an understanding of the person in their context' such that it can deliver 'an integrated whole-person model of healthcare'.[8]

This provides a convenient segue into participants' viewpoints on psy science treatments which, like their opinions on diagnosis, were varied. Experiences with talking therapies were generally described as positive but were found wanting insofar as they did not seem to address the women's sociocultural contexts. The consensus on the efficacy and even appropriateness of pharmacological remedies was less clear, and contrasting views on this were sometimes held simultaneously by the same participant—recall Farah's uncertainty as to whether Zoloft had helped her and Daniella's ambivalence regarding the efficacy of antidepressants. I am also reminded of how Ellen and Olivia alluded to the chemical imbalance model in describing how antidepressants had mitigated their mental distress; both also displayed astute insight into how exogenous conditions and gendered socialisation were strongly implicated in their social anxiety.

How best to proceed in aiding women experiencing mental distress, of which social anxiety is but one form, depends on how Utopian a vision one might be willing to entertain. I for one would be in favour of a social model of care which embraces different ways of being.[9] Another, parallel, avenue would be the adoption of a lateral model of support for those experiencing acute emotional distress or crisis—the most renowned of these alternative services is R. D. Laing's therapeutic community Kingsley Hall, which operated between 1965 and 1970.[10] Judi Chamberlin, in her book *On Our Own*, writes in depth on other alternatives to mental institutions: voluntary, peer-run services in which people are not cleaved into 'sick' and 'healthy', but within which individuals can find support from those who have gone through similar experiences. Although at first glance, such institutions might not seem germane to the topic of this book—experiencing social anxiety is seldom grounds to deem somebody as being 'at risk of harm to themselves or others',[11] and thus eligible for being 'sectioned'. But I remind the reader of participants' narratives on delayed help-seeking and that *all* of them had experienced other forms of mental distress—intense sadness, severe restriction of food—which were difficult to untangle from their social anxiety. Such services could therefore have utility for women akin to those in my sample.

While extensive discussion of these alternative services is beyond the scope of this book,[12] I wish to draw particular attention to two examples about which Chamberlin writes: Elizabeth Stone House, whose ethos was based on feminism, and the Vancouver Emotional Emergency Center. In keeping with my seeking to contextualise women's SAD in terms of their environment, Chamberlin writes that these alternatives

> [T]ried to make important connections between individual unhappiness and societal conditions [...] focusing particularly on operating effectively as a collective and on the relationship between 'going crazy' and the political and social environment.[13] Making these political connections is essential in developing a true alternative, since it helps to locate the cause of people's distress in the very real pressures of their lives rather than believing that it arises out of some mysterious process.[14]

Chamberlin adds to this by sharing her own experience at the Vancouver Emotional Emergency Center. Most relevant to the preceding chapter, she echoes Laing's remarks about schizophrenia being a 'metanoiac voyage':[15]

> I had followed my pain and fear toward what I thought would be death, and instead I had found a source of life, my own sense of self, which had always been hidden from me. Out of struggle and pain, I had been reborn.[16]

Though I am a proponent of such services, they are few and far between at the time of writing, particularly in the UK. As such, I fear that the move towards a social model of care, and the proliferation of services like those described by Chamberlin, will be painfully slow. In the interests of immediacy, our best hope might therefore lie in critical psychiatry which,[17] beginning in the 1990s, could be described as a successor of the anti-psychiatry movement. Critical psychiatry's essential position is described by founding member of the Critical Psychiatry Network, Duncan Double, in stating that 'functional mental illness should not be reduced to brain disease'.[18] The Network represents the application of key ideas on which this book is premised within the constraints of mainstream psychiatry. That is, on the one hand, the Network distances itself from the absolutist strands of Thomas S. Szasz's work which deny 'mental illness'. On the other hand, while not opposed to the use of psychotropic medication, the Network adopts a sceptical approach, echoing my critique of biological psychiatry and the pharmaceutical industry from Chap. 2.

Perhaps most significant to the approach taken by this book, the Network focuses 'on understanding the person and why they have presented with the problems they have in the context of their life situation'.[19] This has much in common with a social approach to mental distress, as outlined by Jerry Tew, which

> [A]ims to see a person *in relationship with* their social and cultural context, rather than seeking to abstract a specific symptom or disease entity that can be treated in isolation. Their wider social situation and their inner experiences are equally important – and inextricably linked.[20]

Given that this book seeks to understand women's social anxiety within their sociocultural context, it aligns with Tew's vision as well as the mission of the Critical Psychiatry Network. As such, this book provides insight for critical psychiatrists seeking to improve the lives of women presenting with distress arising from, giving rise to, or in any way associated with, social anxiety.

In suggesting this, however, it is important to note that I am not seeking to 'cure' women who have these experiences. Rather, I find immense utility in Tew's concept of 'recovery', which

> [E]merged from the experiences of those who have gone through mental distress. It shifts the emphasis from a medical discourse of symptom reduction to a more holistic perspective in which 'recovery' is seen as a journey of discovery and empowerment in which people reclaim valued identities and social roles, irrespective of whether they may continue to have certain unusual mental or emotional experiences. It also focuses on people's strengths and resources, rather than having a preoccupation with their 'deficits' and what they may (temporarily) be unable to do.[21]

Tew's model of recovery thus meshes well with a more lateral model of support, of which Chamberlin's alternative services are emblematic. Marrying this with an approach which heeds the cultural milieu in which women find themselves, I echo Sasha Claire McInnes's call for 'ethical, responsive, choice-oriented, label[-]free mental health supports for women' and 'much more feminist thinking and action in the context of the emotional lives of women, mental health policy and practice'.[22]

Since McInnes's tenets advocate for feminist approaches to women's mental distress, it is timely to revisit the epistemological position underpinning this book, namely feminist standpoint theory. This is concerned with bringing about social change and empowering women: ends which, Jane M. Ussher tells us, can be achieved by focussing 'on women's agency and by providing new accounts of women's experience'.[23] This book's providing a space for socially anxious women to define SAD for themselves and talk about their experiences thus concords with the aims which Ussher outlines.

Furthermore, Ussher makes the argument that in listening to women, research can 'challenge the status quo and [...] provide the material to bring about change'.[24] As per Ussher's argument, this book's forging an alternative narrative on women's SAD brings to light considerations for mental health professionals and policymakers seeking to improve the lives of socially anxious women. But it is not only socially anxious women who stand to gain. Kimberlé Crenshaw contends that collective action and avoiding the compartmentalisation of experiences along single axes of oppression is achieved by 'placing those who currently are marginalized in the center'. In turn, through 'restructuring and remaking the world where necessary', it is not only the most disadvantaged, but also the singularly disadvantaged who might garner benefit:[25] perhaps women who *do not* identify with the SAD diagnosis, in this case. For, as Susie Orbach draws our attention to the 'painful continuity between most women's daily experience and that of the anorectic woman',[26] there seems also to be a continuity between most women's daily experience and that of the *socially anxious* woman. Some of the women I interviewed even drew attention to this themselves—think about Ria's account of her sister's need for external validation, or Ellen's view that her appearance anxieties likely extended to most women.

In the spirit of Crenshaw's call for collectivity, Caplan proposes that 'friendship, consciousness-raising groups, and social action might be more appropriate than therapy for dealing with forms of oppression as they lack the stigma of a diagnosis'.[27] I thus see the exchange of ideas and experiences among socially anxious women—akin to a revival of second-wave feminism's consciousness-raising groups—as being instrumental in alleviating their mental distress. For one, it would facilitate the interrogation of the extent to which women's sociocultural milieu is conducive to their experiences of social anxiety. In turn, it could help them to see that their problems are not as unique to them as they might have thought.

Chamberlin also advocates for the importance of consciousness-raising groups for ex-mental patients, alluding to their being an inversion of psychiatric treatments—treatments which are predicated on problems being individual as opposed to societal. She argues that

> Consciousness raising [...] helps people to see that their so-called symptoms are indications of real problems [...] Instead of believing that they have a defect in their psychic makeup (or neurochemical system), participants learn to recognize the oppressive conditions in their daily lives.[28]

And, in keeping with anti-psychiatry, Chamberlin makes the case that

> Many of the experiences people have had become comprehensible when they are not hidden by psychiatric language. I have seen people in consciousness-raising groups make the exciting discovery that they can draw meaning from what had been dismissed as 'hallucinations' or 'delusions.'[29]

This section finds a fitting end in the words of novelist Alice Walker, for she tells us that one must 'resist the temptation to think what afflicts you is peculiar to you. Have faith that what is in your consciousness can be communicated to the consciousness of all. And is, in many cases, already there'.[30]

Remit and Future Directions

As I noted at the commencement of Chap. 3, although my small sample *is* diverse, there are nonetheless voices which are not as well represented as I would have ideally liked. These include youth (16–24), older women, and women under the LGBTQIA+ umbrella. As such, engaging with the narratives of socially anxious women from these sociodemographic groups would be an extremely important avenue for future research.

In further demarcating the remit of this book, I want to draw on Orbach, who delimits the scope of her writing on women's eating problems by noting that 'the overwhelming evidence' for these problems' aetiologies lies 'in the direction of social and psychological explanations'.[31] She chooses not to entertain biomedical theories since she argues that they cannot account for 'the rise in anorexia, the incidence of episodic bulimia and the Western cultural obsession with thinness'.[32] In a similar manner, I have distanced myself from biological and evolutionary accounts of women's SAD, which often rely on implicit sexism. Furthermore, these models give no attention to the impact of postfeminist and neoliberal discourses which demand continuous self-betterment; the imperative for women to adhere to (often contradictory) gender role expectations, no matter the cost to their wellbeing; and the myriad social factors which the women I interviewed cited as contributors to their social anxiety. Instead, this book develops a holistic, embodied account of how women experience social anxiety in twenty-first-century Britain.

I find another key remark in the writings of Orbach, for she states that 'psychological symptoms express the ideas a culture has at any given time about itself'.[33] I therefore wonder what the narratives of the women in this book can reveal to this end. Perhaps they tell us that our culture prizes being 'normal'; it mandates cultivating a particular type of body and subjectivity; and the neoliberal, postfeminist individualism with which it is replete reaches right into our minds, for mental distress is construed as very much an individual problem. As feminist scholar and activist Silvia Federici once said of women's socialisation: 'If you don't like it, it is your problem, your failure, your guilt, and your abnormality.'[34]

But our culture at the time of writing concerns me for a further reason. Its increasing move to medicalise, and medicate, sees a withering of its tolerance of different emotions and ways of being. Caplan articulates this in describing how '[w]e live in a technologically[-]oriented society in which we are urged to treat every feeling other than happiness as mental illness so that there can be a quick fix, usually with medication'.[35] Simon J. Williams is also critical of the dominant perspective that emotions are 'failures in instrumental reasoning' and posits that a world without them would be 'a dull, empty affair without doubt'.[36] To quote Christopher Lane, the sad consequence of 'mood brightening' and treating personality traits as medical issues 'is a vast, perhaps unrecoverable, loss of emotional range, an impoverishment of human experience'.[37] That is not to say that women who experience social anxiety as distressing should not seek help. Rather, I am worried by our society's move towards 'cauteriz[ing] pain' and 'averting any incident that would give us even a foretaste of it'.[38] In the words of psychiatrist Viktor Frankl, '[S]uffering is not always a pathological phenomenon; rather than being a symptom of neurosis, suffering may well be a human achievement.'[39] On this point, Tew proposes that

> [E]xpressions of mental distress are ways in which we may be trying to express 'the meaning of our lives'.[40] So, instead of writing them off as 'symptoms' of a 'mental illness', distress experiences should be respected and taken seriously as an attempt to communicate something – perhaps about an injustice or a 'problem of living' – which may be very hard to express by more conventional means.[41]

Applying this to social anxiety, Susie Scott cites a web resource on shyness which presents 'exploring shy feelings as a means of "finding the real you" and reaching a deeper understanding of the self'.[42] Most pertinent for the perspective endorsed by this book, Scott notes that 'the idea that we can achieve personal growth by surviving psychological distress reminds us of Laing's influential remarks about schizophrenia as a voyage of self-discovery, and suggests that shyness represents a more "authentic" mode of being'.[43] Our social anxiety might therefore have much to tell us not only about our culture but about ourselves—if only we let it.

As to what else women's experiences of social anxiety might tell us, the preceding chapters touched upon several themes, the full exploration of which was not possible within the confines of this book. I will visit these in turn and suggest how future research might build upon them.

An unexpected finding was the resonance between participants' narratives and the Dissociative Disorders: Dissociative Identity Disorder (DID) and, to a lesser extent, Depersonalization/Derealization Disorder. To make sense of this, I drew on Meg-John Barker's work on 'plurality', wherein they frame multiple selves as another way of being. Barker makes brief mention of psychiatry's classification of what used to be called 'Multiple Personality Disorder' and its representation in the media: that is, often very negative and involving criminality. Barker's own experience of plurality stands in contradistinction to this, since they view their multiple selves positively. Farah's perspective on her social anxiety was analogous, for she remarked, 'Maybe it's not a bad thing if I have this experience.' Since my aim throughout this work has been to reframe and critique psychiatric discourses on SAD, a corresponding approach would be apt for exploring the gendered nature of plurality; engaging with the narratives of women (self-)diagnosed with DID, and providing a corrective to psychiatric and popular discourses on multiple selves.

A further diagnosis which drew links with participants' accounts was that of autism, particularly autistic women's accounts of wearing a 'mask'[44] or 'pretending to be normal'[45]—recall Phoebe's description of mimicking her sister when socialising; Farah's strategy of adopting a mask to cover her shyness; and Daniella's experience of 'put[ting] up a face'. Extant research has explored the sociological and cultural factors shaping women's lower rates of ASD diagnosis,[46] including gender bias in diagnostic criteria;[47] autism's misdiagnosis with psychiatric diagnoses; and its 'co-morbidities'—notably, social anxiety.[48] Future research might follow this book's blueprint to engage with autistic women's narratives. In so doing, it could provide a corrective to current diagnostic criteria's masculine bias and unearth how normative white femininity shapes the experiences of autistic women.

As 'co-morbidities', psychiatric diagnoses and otherwise, have formed a backdrop to this book, another recurring theme has been social media. This seemed to augment social anxiety for some of the women I interviewed, such as Ellen and Ria. Perhaps an unconscious awareness of this exacerbatory potential has underpinned my own eschewing of all social media. When I pull this thread, I find that imagining my avatar existing somewhere *out there* puts me incredibly ill at ease. This nebulous image of me is however also tangible insofar as it can be played and replayed, chopped and changed, evaluated and re-evaluated. It is therefore simultaneously free-floating and indelibly marked in cyberspace. What is more, I feel powerless to control others' assessments of it—which, of course, are publicly quantified by views, shares, likes, and follows. By comparison, it seems a small mercy that in real life there are only others' real-time impressions and memories of me about which I fret. The thin line of acceptable femininity is tricky enough to walk in the flesh: attempting to manage a digital extension of myself that must also strike this fine balance, and to do so *without* experiencing social anxiety, has to be a fool's errand.

While social media seemed to stoke several participants' social anxiety, some of their remarks left me wondering whether it could be used more constructively. In particular, Ellen mentioned rejecting mainstream social media: she proposed unfollowing Instagram influencers and engaging with the body positivity movement online. In following this proposal through, the feelings of inadequacy that women like Ellen experience at the hands of mainstream social media might be superseded by a more positive body image and less distress about others' perceptions.

In addition to the above, social media could provide a vehicle for consciousness-raising which was not available to our forebears, and I daresay the online version of this might prove more palatable for the socially anxious woman. There is also the advantage of relative anonymity—consider the Reddit community 'social anxiety'.[49] This is but one example which would fit the bill in providing a viable means of communication with other socially anxious women: a technological spin on the groups established by our second-wave sisters. Further work might therefore ask the obverse of what this book has argued with respect to social media: can it be used to alleviate women's social anxiety and, if so, how?

Personal Reflections

In writing this book, I have aligned myself with a tenet of psychologists Mary Crawford and Jeanne Marecek: that the research process should be 'one of mutual collaboration in which the research participant is acknowledged as the primary interpreter of her or his experience and the research initiator is acknowledged as emotionally involved and as changed by the process of doing the research'.[50] In rendering the voices of participants central, acknowledging my own positionality, and adopting a reflexive approach, I have met the first two of Crawford and Marecek's criteria. What remains is the question of whether I have been changed by the research process.

Firstly, I have come to realise that, when confronted with a research question, the most satisfactory and nuanced explanation is often, in the words of Marion Milner, 'a marriage between the two protagonists, not an either/or solution'.[51] I have evidenced this merging in drawing on the work of anti-psychiatrists, philosophers, psychologists, psychotherapists, social workers, psychoanalysts, feminist scholars, medical doctors, journalists, sociologists, and psychiatrists alike in formulating my alternative narrative on women's SAD.

Most importantly, it is through listening to the stories of socially anxious women that I have come to realise that their anguish, and perhaps mine too, is manifold. For one, we deal with the distress, of which social anxiety is part, resulting from how society treats us by dint of our non-normativity. Our distress is then compounded by the compulsion we feel not only to conceal our non-normativity, but to conceal our resulting distress. And, at least for me, social anxiety is nigh impossible to hide. In the case of socially anxious women then, the following words from Albert Camus encapsulate our experience rather well: 'Nobody realizes that some people expend tremendous energy merely to be normal.'[52]

Notes

1. E.g. Jane M. Ussher, 'Premenstrual Syndrome: Reconciling Disciplinary Divides through the Adoption of a Material-discursive Epistemological Standpoint', *Annual Review of Sex Research*, 7.1 (1996), 218–51 https://doi.org/10.1080/10532528.1996.10559914 p. 235.
   Elizabeth Mollard, 'Exploring Paradigms in Postpartum Depression Research: The Need for Feminist Pragmatism', *Health Care for Women International*, 36.4 (2015), 378–91 https://doi.org/10.1080/07399332.2014.903951
   Tamara Kayali Browne, 'Is Premenstrual Dysphoric Disorder Really a Disorder?' *Journal of Bioethical Inquiry*, 12.2 (2015), 313–30 https://doi.org/10.1007/s11673-014-9567-7
   Natasha Mauthner, 'Towards a Feminist Understanding of Postnatal Depression', *Feminism and Psychology*, 3.3 (1993), 350–55 https://doi.org/10.1177/0959353593033006
   Chloë Taylor, 'Female Sexual Dysfunction, Feminist Sexology, and the Psychiatry of the Normal', *Feminist Studies*, 41.2 (2015), 259–92 https://doi.org/10.15767/feministstudies.41.2.259
2. Michel Foucault, *The Will to Knowledge, The History of Sexuality: I*, trans. Robert Hurley (Harmondsworth: Penguin, 1998), p. 101.
3. Michael R. Liebowitz, Jack M. Gorman, Abby J. Fyer, and Donald F. Klein, 'Social Phobia: Review of a Neglected Anxiety Disorder', *Archives of General Psychiatry*, 42.7 (1985), 729–36 https://doi.org/10.1001/archpsyc.1985.01790300097013
4. Paula J. Caplan, *When Jonny and Jane Come Marching Home: How All of Us Can Help Veterans* (Hanover, NH: Scribl, 2019), p. 40.

5. I refer interested readers to a journal article in which I discuss this facet of participants' narratives in greater depth. See Katie Masters, 'Women's Experiences of Social Anxiety Disorder: Privileging Marginalised Perspectives and Rewriting Dominant Narratives', *International Mad Studies Journal*, 1.1 (2022), e1–21 https://doi.org/10.58544/imsj.v1i1.5244
6. Sami Timimi, 'No More Psychiatric Labels: Why Formal Psychiatric Diagnostic Systems Should Be Abolished', *International Journal of Clinical and Health Psychology*, 14.3 (2014), 208–15 https://doi.org/10.1016/j.ijchp.2014.03.004 p. 213.
7. Ibid.
8. Ibid.
9. For further discussion of different ways of being and social anxiety, see Masters, 'Women's Experiences of Social Anxiety Disorder'.
10. Adrian Chapman, 'Dwelling in Strangeness: Accounts of the Kingsley Hall Community, London (1965–1970), Established by R. D. Laing', *Journal of Medical Humanities*, 42.3 (2021), 471–94 https://doi.org/10.1007/s10912-020-09656-0
11. This is the criterion for involuntary detention ('sectioning') in the UK as per the Mental Health Act (1983). See NHS, *Mental Health Act* (2022) https://www.nhs.uk/mental-health/social-care-and-your-rights/mental-health-and-the-law/mental-health-act/ [accessed 29 March 2023].
12. For more on alternative services, see Judi Chamberlin, *On Our Own: Patient-controlled Alternatives to the Mental Health System* (Lawrence, Massachusetts: National Empowerment Centre, Inc., 2012[1977]), pp. 161–62.
13. Personal interview with David Myers by Judi Chamberlin, December 20, 1976.
14. Chamberlin, *On Our Own*, p. 156.
15. R. D. Laing, 'Metanoia: Some Experiences at Kingsley Hall, London', in *Going Crazy: The Radical Therapy of R. D. Laing and Others*, ed. by Hendrik M. Ruitenbeek (New York, Bantam Books, 1972), p. 12.
16. Chamberlin, *On Our Own*, p. 67.
17. Hugh Middleton and Joanna Moncrieff, 'Critical Psychiatry: A Brief Overview', *BJPsych Advances*, 25.1 (2019), 47–54 https://doi.org/10.1192/bja.2018.38
18. Duncan Double, 'Twenty Years of the Critical Psychiatry Network', *The British Journal of Psychiatry*, 214.2 (2019), 61–62 https://doi.org/10.1192/bjp.2018.181 p. 61.
19. Ibid., p. 62.
20. Jerry Tew, *Social Approaches to Mental Distress* (Basingstoke: Palgrave Macmillan, 2011), p. 16.

21. Ibid., p. 12.
22. Sasha Claire McInnes, 'The Political is Personal – Or, why Have a Revolution (from within or without) when You Can Have Soma?' *Feminist Review*, 68.1 (2001), 160–66 https://doi.org/10.1080/01417780110042455 p. 165.
23. Sandra Harding, 'Rethinking Standpoint Epistemology: "What is Strong Objectivity?"' in *Feminist Epistemologies*, ed. by Linda Martín Alcoff and Elizabeth Potter (London: Routledge, 1993), 63–78.
    C. Swann, 'Psychology and Self[-]reported PMS: An Evaluation of Different Research Strategies' (unpublished doctoral thesis, University of London, 1996).
    All cited in Jane M. Ussher, 'Premenstrual Syndrome: Fact, Fantasy, or Fiction?', in *Psychology at the Turn of the Millennium. Vol. 2: Social, Developmental and Clinical Perspectives*, ed. by Lars Backman and Claes von Hofsten (New York: Psychology Press, 2002), 497–528, p. 521.
24. Ibid.
25. Kimberlé Crenshaw, 'Demarginalizing the Intersection of Race and Sex: A Black Feminist Critique of Antidiscrimination Doctrine, Feminist Theory and Antiracist Politics', *University of Chicago Legal Forum*, 1.8 (1989), 139–67 http://chicagounbound.uchicago.edu/uclf/vol1989/iss1/8 p. 167.
26. Susie Orbach, *Hunger Strike: Starving amidst Plenty* (London and New York: Karnac, 2005), p. 78.
27. Carl C. Bell, 'They Say You're Crazy: How the World's Most Powerful Psychiatrists Decide Who's Normal' [Book Review], *JAMA*, 274.20 (1995), 1639 https://doi.org/10.1001/jama.1995.03530200077048 p. 1639.
28. Chamberlin, *On Our Own*, p. 71.
29. Ibid., p. 188.
30. Alice Walker, *The Temple of my Familiar* (San Diego: Harcourt, Brace, Jovanovich, 1989), p. 317.
31. Orbach, *Hunger Strike*, p. 162.
32. Ibid.
33. Ibid., p. 47.
34. Silvia Federici, *Wages against Housework* (London: Power of Women Collective, 1975), p. 3.
35. Caplan, *When Jonny and Jane Come Marching Home*, p. 13.
36. Simon J. Williams, 'Reason, Emotion and Embodiment: Is "Mental" Health a Contradiction in Terms?', *Sociology of Health and Illness*, 22.5 (2000), 559–81 https://doi.org/10.1111/1467-9566.00220 p. 562.
37. Lane, *Shyness: How Normal Behavior Became a Sickness* (Yale University Press, 2007) https://ebookcentral.proquest.com/lib/bham/reader.action?docID=3420940 [accessed 6 January 2021] p. 8.

38. Ibid., p. 170.
39. Viktor E. Frankl. *Man's Search for Meaning: An Introduction to Logotherapy* (London: Hodder and Stoughton, 1978[1964]), p. 104.
40. Anne E. Plumb, 'New Mental Health Legislation. A Lifesaver? Changing Paradigm and Practice', *Social Work Education*, 18.4 (1999), 459–78 https://doi.org/10.1080/02615479911220441 p. 471.
41. Jerry Tew, *Social Approaches to Mental Distress*, p. 16.
42. Shy and Free, *Shyness Self-help How-to* (2004) http://www.shyandfree.com [accessed 27 July 2004] cited in Susie Scott, 'The Medicalisation of Shyness: From Social Misfits to Social Fitness', *Sociology of Health and Illness*, 28.2 (2006), 133–53 https://doi.org/10.1111/j.1467-9566.2006.00485.x p. 148.
43. Ronald David Laing, *The Politics of Experience and the Bird of Paradise* (Harmondsworth: Penguin, 1967), cited in Scott, 'The Medicalisation of Shyness', p. 148.
44. National Autistic Society, *How Do Women and Girls Experience Autism?* (2018) https://www.autism.org.uk/about/what-is/gender/stories.aspx [accessed 31 July 2020].
45. Sarah Bargiela, Robyn Steward, and William Mandy, 'The Experiences of Late-diagnosed Women with Autism Spectrum Conditions: An Investigation of the Female Autism Phenotype', *Journal of Autism and Developmental Disorders*, 46.10 (2016), 3281–94 https://doi.org/10.1007/s10803-016-2872-8
46. Liane Holliday Willey, *Pretending To Be Normal: Living with Asperger's Syndrome* (London/Philadelphia: Jessica Kingsley Publishers, 2015).
    Rudy Simone, *Aspergirls* (London/Philadelphia: Jessica Kingsley Publishers, 2010).
47. Jolynn L. Haney, 'Autism, Females, and the DSM-5: Gender Bias in Autism Diagnosis', *Social Work in Mental Health*, 14. 4 (2016), 396–407 https://doi.org/10.1080/15332985.2015.1031858
48. Sarah Hendrickx, *Women and Girls with Autism Spectrum Disorder* (London/Philadelphia: Jessica Kingsley Publishers, 2015).
49. Reddit, *Social Anxiety* (n.d.) https://www.reddit.com/r/socialanxiety/ [accessed 27 September 2020].
50. Mary Crawford and Jeanne Marecek, 'Psychology Reconstructs the Female: 1968–1988', *Psychology of Women Quarterly*, 13.2 (1989), 147–65 https://doi.org/10.1111/j.1471-6402.1989.tb00993.x p. 159.
51. Marion Milner, *A Life of One's Own* (Taylor and Francis Group, 2011) https://ebookcentral.proquest.com/lib/bham/reader.action?docID=672403 [accessed 24 September 2020] p. 178.
52. Albert Camus, *Notebooks, 1942–1951* [*Carnets, Janvier 1942 – Mars 1951*] trans. Justin O'Brien (Chicago: Ivan R. Dee, 2010), p. 80.

Index[1]

[1] Note: Page numbers followed by 'n' refer to notes.

K. Masters, *Feminist and Anti-Psychiatry Perspectives on 'Social Anxiety Disorder'*,
https://doi.org/10.1007/978-3-031-48707-1

R

T

SPRINGER NATURE

GPSR Compliance

The European Union's (EU) General Product Safety Regulation (GPSR) is a set of rules that requires consumer products to be safe and our obligations to ensure this.

If you have any concerns about our products, you can contact us on ProductSafety@springernature.com

In case Publisher is established outside the EU, the EU authorized representative is:

Springer Nature Customer Service Center GmbH
Europaplatz 3
69115 Heidelberg, Germany

FSC
www.fsc.org
MIX
Papier | Fördert gute Waldnutzung
FSC® C083411

Kolibri 360 GmbH
Ferdinand-Jühlke-Straße 7
99095 Erfurt, Deutschland
produktsicherheit@kolibri360.de